The Lies We Eat

DAVID W. BROWN

THE LIES WE EAT

This book is dedicated to you—the readers who have chosen to take charge of your health before a crisis demands it. Your willingness to act today is not only the greatest gift you can give yourself, but also a profound act of love toward those who depend on you. It is also dedicated to those already facing serious health challenges. Please know that hope is never lost. Every positive step, no matter how small, can open the door to healing and renewal.

To each person holding this book: may these pages inspire, encourage, and empower you to create lasting health, restore balance, and reclaim your life.

Disclaimer

"I am not a doctor, but I have dedicated many years to researching the impact of a plant-based diet on cancer and exploring the harmful chemical processes that can affect our health. The information provided in this book is supported by scientific studies, all of which are available on thep53.com website for those who have purchased the book. While I do not offer personalized medical advice, I share insights from research studies and the conclusions drawn by scientists in the field. Not all doctors are aligned with or influenced by the pharmaceutical industry. Many are compassionate professionals dedicated to helping their patients live healthier lives. In fact, I have personally shared research with physicians who recognize and support the very truths presented in this book. A plant-based diet has been shown to contribute to the reversal of certain cancers and other health conditions, and it may reduce the risk of developing certain cancers, as supported by the cited studies. Stories in this book illustrate how nutrition science applies to real life. They are composites based on research and clinical experience, not individual medical cases. To access the full list of references, please email proof of purchase to dave@thep53.com, and you will be given login credentials to view the sources used in this book."

David W. Brown

Foreword

When I first came across Dave Brown's work, I didn't realize just how much it would change my life. As a life coach, I've always been deeply invested in helping people create lasting transformation. But when it came to health, I often felt like something was missing. My clients could work on mindset, productivity, and relationships, but if they didn't have energy, if their health was deteriorating, everything else suffered.

That's when I discovered the **P53 Diet & Lifestyle** — not just as a book, but as a philosophy for living. What struck me immediately was that it wasn't just another diet fad. It wasn't built on gimmicks, shortcuts, or industry-driven myths. Instead, it was grounded in **decades of research, real science, and lived experience**. Dave had done the hard work — digging into how nutrition, lifestyle, and the body's own healing systems all connect.

I decided to put it to the test in my own life. And the results were undeniable. I experienced improvements in energy, focus, and vitality that no supplement or trendy diet had ever given me. The truth is simple: the body wants to heal, and when you give it what it needs — real, whole plant foods — it responds.

But what made the deepest impression on me wasn't just how the **P53 Diet** worked for me personally. It was watching Dave in action. I've had the privilege of going with him as he consults with people battling cancer and other serious ailments. I've sat in with Dave as families were desperate for hope. I've listened as Dave explained — calmly, passionately, and clearly

— how food, lifestyle, and small daily choices can reshape the body's terrain.

I've watched people light up as they realized that they weren't powerless. That healing wasn't only in the hands of doctors or pills. That their plate could be their medicine. And I've watched many of those same people make changes — eating differently, moving differently, thinking differently — and experience transformations they never thought possible.

It's one thing to read about nutrition in an abstract way. It's another to watch it **change lives in real time.** That's what I've seen over and over again walking alongside Dave.

That's also why I decided to take my learning even deeper by enrolling in **P53 University**, to become a certified plant-based nutrition specialist. For me, this isn't just about improving my own health anymore — it's about helping others. And I couldn't think of a better teacher or mentor than Dave Brown. I looked at a lot of other nutrition courses before choosing P53 University, but none came close to the depth this program offers. I'll be honest — I about pulled my hair out going through the biochemistry section — but that's exactly what makes it different. This isn't one of those quick weekend certifications. The knowledge I'm gaining through P53 University is giving me the strongest tools possible to truly help other people.

Because here's the truth: behind this book lies not just research, but **years of passion and commitment.** Dave has poured himself into studying nutrition from every angle. He's read the studies, examined the evidence, challenged the myths, and refused to accept the convenient answers that industries feed us. More importantly, he's put that knowledge into practice — both in his own life and in the lives of others.

That's what makes this new book, **The Lies We Eat: The Truth That Heals,** so powerful. It distills years of research, experience, and truth-telling into a format that anyone can pick up and understand. It takes the complex science that Dave has written about in his other books — **The P53 Diet & Lifestyle, How You Are Being Poisoned, Understanding Hormones, Enzymes & Cell Receptors,** and **Taste Versus Cancer** — and simplifies it into something that's clear, direct, and immediately actionable.

And perhaps most importantly, it **exposes the myths**.

These lies have been repeated so often that they've become accepted as truth. But when you peel back the marketing, the science tells a very different story.

This book doesn't just give information. It gives **tools**. Every chapter ends with Key Takeaways, Action Steps, and a Closing Message — so the truths you read don't just stay on the page, they move into your daily life.

I believe that's what sets Dave apart. He doesn't just want you to know the science. He wants you to **live the change**. He wants you to taste the difference, feel the energy, experience the healing — and then, like me, share it with others.

As a life coach, I've always believed that transformation begins when people reclaim their power. And there's no area where that's more true than health. Reading this book, you'll discover that you don't have to be a victim of genetics, industry lies, or chronic disease. You are in control. You always have been.

I'm honored not only to write this foreword, but to continue learning, teaching, and sharing as part of the P53 mission. And I'm grateful to Dave for his years of tireless research, his clarity of teaching, and his compassion for people who desperately need truth.

So as you turn these pages, remember: this isn't just another book on health. It's a guide, a roadmap, and a wake-up call. Read it with an open mind. Let it challenge what you've been taught. And most importantly, put it into action.

Because health isn't complicated. It's not hidden in a pill or a supplement. It's on your plate, in your habits, and in your hands.

And as Dave always reminds me: **the truth heals.**

Truett Standefer
Life Coach
lumen8life.com

Introduction

Health is supposed to be simple. For most of human history, it was. We ate food that grew from the earth. We moved daily, rested deeply, and lived in harmony with the cycles of nature. Our bodies knew how to thrive, repair, and heal themselves.

But in the modern world, health has been stolen. Confusing marketing, toxic foods, and a culture built on pills and quick fixes have left millions of people sick, tired, and searching for answers. Doctors prescribe more drugs, companies sell more supplements, and the average person feels less and less in control of their own body.

This book was written to flip that story. Its purpose is simple: to show you that **you are in control of your health**. Not the pharmaceutical industry. Not the food industry. Not even the medical system. You are in control. Unlike my other books, which explore the science in detail, this one keeps things simple and easy to follow.

The Roots of This Book

Over the years, I've written several books that dig deep into the science behind disease, nutrition, and healing. Each has its place, but together they form the foundation of this summary-style book you now hold.

· In **The P53 Diet & Lifestyle**, I explained how the foods we eat and the way we live directly impact the "guardian of the genome" — the P53 protein that protects us against cancer and disease. That book showed how lifestyle choices can literally flip the switch between health and illness.

- In ***How You Are Being Poisoned***, I pulled back the curtain on the everyday toxins — pesticides, food additives, dyes, pollutants, even medications — that slowly chip away at health.
- In ***Understanding Hormones, Enzymes & Cell Receptors***, I broke down how the body actually works on a cellular level — how hormones send signals, how enzymes spark reactions, and how cell receptors decide whether healing or harm takes place.
- In ***Taste Versus Cancer***, I showed how the very foods we eat can either fuel cancer or fight it. It wasn't abstract science — it was a call to arms, showing how plants defend us while animal products and processed junk feed disease.

Each of those books is a deep dive. This one is different. Here, I bring all of that work together in a way that's simple, accessible, and designed for anyone to understand.

Beyond the Books: A Bigger Movement

But my work has never been just about writing books. It's about building a movement that puts power back into people's hands.

That's why I created the **P53 Diet site** — an online hub where anyone can learn the basics of plant-based eating, recipes, meal planning, and start taking immediate steps toward better health. It's a place where the science of food becomes practical in everyday life.

It's also why I founded **P53 University** — an educational platform for those who want to go deeper, to study plant-based nutrition in detail, and even become certified to teach others.

It's not about selling degrees. It's about raising up leaders who can carry this message into their communities.

And it's why we launched **P53 Food Carts** — bringing healthy, plant-based meals directly into neighborhoods. For too long, "fast food" has meant fried, processed, and harmful. Our carts prove that fast can also mean fresh, healing, and life-giving.

Why This Book Matters Now

We live in a crisis of misinformation. Big Food sells junk with "healthy" labels. Big Pharma pushes pills for every symptom. Supplement companies market powders as if they can replace real food.

The result? A world where the average person is overfed but undernourished. Where diseases that were once rare are now common. Where people believe health is something you buy in a bottle, not something you build with a plate.

This book exists to cut through the noise. Not with jargon, but with clarity.

What You'll Learn

Inside, you'll discover why nutrient deficiencies are everywhere, how animal products fuel disease, why processed fats and sugars rob you of energy, and how whole plants rebuild health. You'll see the truth about pills, supplements, toxins, and food labels. You'll learn how exercise, habits, and lifestyle choices reshape your terrain and give your body what it has always wanted — the chance to heal.

Every chapter offers not just information, but practical steps you can start immediately.

The Promise of Simplicity

If you've read my other books, you know I don't shy away from science. But this book is different. It's about seeing the whole picture in plain language.

Think of it as the "essentials" version of everything I've ever taught — the one you can hand to a friend or family member who doesn't want a textbook, but who needs the truth.

Taking Back Control

At its core, this book is about reclaiming what's yours: your health, your energy, your life. It's about understanding that the most powerful medicine isn't sold in a pharmacy or a supplement shop. It's grown in soil. It's cooked in your kitchen. It's lived out in your daily habits.

Health is not complicated. It is not expensive. And it is not out of reach.

The truth is simple: **you are in control. Always have been. Always will be.**

Please visit thep53.com for more info.

The

P

53

University

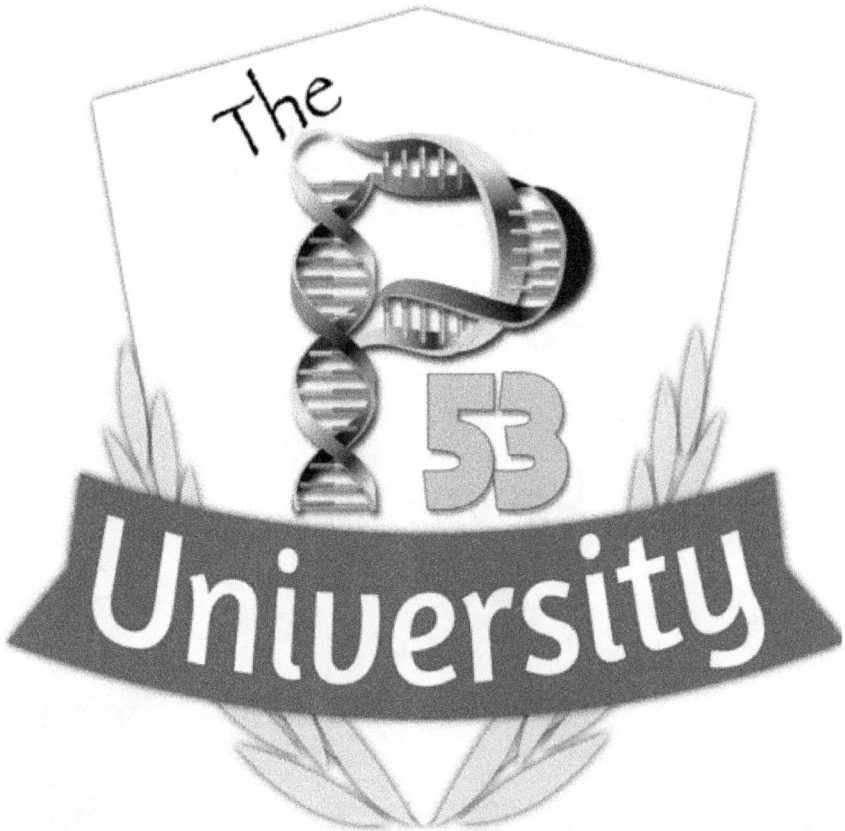

Give a Free Radical a Home...

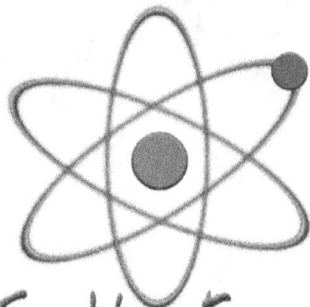

Eat Your Fruit

thep53.com

Contents

Chapter 1

Nutrient Deficiencies: The Silent Epidemic

Most people think deficiencies are something that only happen in faraway, impoverished countries — children with bowed legs from rickets, sailors with scurvy on old wooden ships, or images in history books of people wasting away from pellagra. But here's the uncomfortable truth: nutrient deficiencies are everywhere, including here, in wealthy nations with overflowing supermarkets and fast-food restaurants on every corner.

How can that be? How can people surrounded by food — with aisles upon aisles of packaged snacks, frozen meals, and drive-thru "value menus" — still be starving for nutrients?

It's simple: most of our food is empty. Empty calories, empty nutrition, empty of what the body really needs.

The food system has changed more in the last 100 years than in the last 10,000. Our ancestors ate food straight from the land — fruits plucked from trees, vegetables pulled from the ground, beans dried in the sun, grains ground fresh. Compare that to today's diet: highly processed, heavily refined, cooked to death, sprayed with chemicals, shipped across continents, stripped of vitamins, and then "fortified" with synthetic substitutes.

People are eating plenty of calories — in fact, more calories than ever before — but those calories are mostly from sugar, refined grains, cheap oils, and animal products. Energy without nutrients. Fuel without spark plugs.

And the result? Millions of people walk around every day feeling tired, foggy, anxious, inflamed, obese, and sick — without realizing why. They blame age. They blame stress. They blame genetics. But underneath it all, their bodies are running on fumes.

This is the silent epidemic. Not famine in the traditional sense, but a famine hidden beneath abundance. Not hunger of the stomach, but hunger of the cells. And like any epidemic, it spreads quietly, until the consequences become unavoidable.

The Old Deficiencies vs. The New Deficiencies

When people think of deficiencies, they usually picture the classic textbook cases:

- **Scurvy (Vitamin C deficiency):** sailors in the 1700s losing teeth, bleeding gums, and dying after months at sea without citrus.
- **Rickets (Vitamin D deficiency):** children in industrial cities with crooked legs because soot-blocked sunlight kept their bodies from making vitamin D.
- **Pellagra (Niacin deficiency):** rural communities surviving on little more than cornmeal, developing dermatitis, diarrhea, dementia, and eventually death.
- **Beriberi (Thiamine deficiency):** people dependent on polished white rice, suffering heart failure and paralysis.

These diseases haven't disappeared — they still occur — but they're far less common in developed nations. What we face now are the **"new deficiencies"**: subtle, chronic, and often ignored by the medical system until they explode into full-blown disease.

- A man who feels exhausted all the time is told he has depression — but no one checks his vitamin D.
- A woman who struggles with constant migraines is given painkillers — but no one checks her magnesium.
- A child who can't focus in school is tested for ADHD — but no one looks at iron or B vitamins.

Deficiencies today rarely look like dramatic wasting away. Instead, they show up as everyday suffering that most people assume is "normal."

The Abundance Paradox

Here's the paradox: **we live in the most overfed, undernourished era in history.**

- Overfed with calories, sugar, fat, salt, and processed ingredients.
- Undernourished when it comes to the essential vitamins, minerals, and phytonutrients the body needs to run properly.

That's why so many modern diseases are skyrocketing — obesity, diabetes, heart disease, cancer, autoimmune conditions, and dementia. They're not caused only by excess. They're caused by excess of the wrong things combined with deficiency of the right things.

The World Health Organization has identified nutrient deficiencies as one of the leading contributors to global disease burden. Inactivity and processed food may dominate the headlines, but underneath, deficiencies quietly fuel the fire.

And here's what makes this epidemic even more dangerous: it's invisible.

There's no breaking news alert that your body is running low on magnesium. There's no push notification when your vitamin D drops in winter. You won't get a flashing warning light on your forehead if your folate is low.

Instead, your body whispers. Fatigue. Irritability. Poor sleep. Frequent colds. Brain fog. Joint pain. Subtle signs that are easy to brush off — until one day they become something bigger.

Food as a Factory vs. Food as Medicine

To understand how we got here, picture two kitchens.

- The **first kitchen** is your grandmother's garden kitchen: tomatoes ripened on the vine, corn shucked fresh, beans simmered in a pot, greens tossed straight into a salad. Every color, every texture, every flavor — full of natural vitamins and minerals.
- The **second kitchen** is today's industrial food plant: white flour bleached and stripped, sugar refined until it's nothing but crystals, oils extracted with chemicals like hexane, vegetables canned and boiled until their nutrients vanish, then all of it wrapped in plastic and "enriched" with a sprinkle of artificial vitamins.

Which one do you think builds a healthy body? Which one leaves you "full" but empty?

This is the crisis. Food has been turned from medicine into product. And the price we pay isn't just at the checkout counter. It's in our health, our energy, and our lifespan.

What Deficiency Looks Like Today

Nutrient deficiency in the modern world doesn't always show up as the "skin and bones" malnutrition you might see in photographs from famine-stricken regions. More often, it looks like the average person at the office, yawning at 3 p.m., reaching for coffee or an energy drink. It looks like the parent who gets home from work too tired to play with their kids. It looks like the teenager with constant acne, poor sleep, and mood swings.

Deficiencies today are often masked by calories. People are eating enough — sometimes more than enough — but what they're eating is stripped of the very vitamins and minerals their cells need. The result? Subtle, creeping health problems that don't always raise red flags in the doctor's office.

Here are some common deficiency-related symptoms most people brush off as "normal life":

- **Low iron** → fatigue, brain fog, brittle nails, restless legs, shortness of breath.
- **Low magnesium** → muscle cramps, poor sleep, anxiety, high blood pressure, headaches.
- **Low vitamin D** → weakened immunity, bone aches, depression, seasonal affective disorder.
- **Low B vitamins** → nerve tingling, irritability, memory lapses, poor concentration.
- **Low potassium** → heart palpitations, weakness, constipation.
- **Low omega-3 fatty acids** → dry skin, inflammation, mood instability.

· **Low zinc** → slow wound healing, frequent infections, loss of taste or smell.

Millions of people live with these symptoms every day, chalking them up to aging, stress, or "just the way things are." Doctors, pressed for time, often treat the symptom with a pill rather than looking for the underlying nutrient gap.

This is why so many modern conditions have become chronic. Instead of asking **what's missing from the body,** we've learned to suppress the discomfort. Painkillers for headaches, antacids for indigestion, sleeping pills for insomnia, antidepressants for mood, energy drinks for fatigue. Each layer of medication covers the whisper of deficiency with another bandage, while the root cause remains unsolved.

Why We're Deficient

If we live in a land of abundance, why are deficiencies so common? The answer lies in how our food is grown, processed, and consumed.

1. Soil Depletion

Our great-grandparents ate spinach, carrots, corn, and beans grown in nutrient-rich soil. Today, industrial farming prioritizes yield over quality. Crops are bred for size, shelf life, and transportability — not nutrition.

Decades of intensive monocropping, chemical fertilizers, and pesticide use have stripped the soil of minerals like magnesium, zinc, and selenium. Without replenishment, the plants that grow in that soil can't absorb what isn't there.

A head of broccoli in 1950 might have contained **twice the calcium and magnesium** of a head of broccoli today. The USDA has quietly documented this nutrient decline, but most people have never heard about it. We still eat vegetables — but they're not the same vegetables our ancestors thrived on.

2. Food Processing

Consider wheat. In its natural form, it contains fiber, B vitamins, magnesium, and healthy fats. But once it's milled into white flour, nearly all of that is stripped away. What's left is starch — empty carbohydrate. The industry response? Add back a sprinkle of synthetic vitamins and call it "enriched." But enrichment never restores the full complexity of what was lost.

Sugar is even worse. Pure sucrose contains zero nutrients beyond calories. It robs the body further by requiring magnesium, zinc, and B vitamins to metabolize. Every spoonful doesn't just fail to nourish you — it drains your reserves.

Then there are oils. Vegetable oils like corn, soybean, and canola are extracted with chemical solvents, bleached, and deodorized. The result is a product that's calorically dense but nutritionally bankrupt.

3. Animal Foods Crowd Out Plants

Meat and dairy are calorie-dense, but compared to fruits, vegetables, legumes, and seeds, they're nutrient-poor. Worse, high intake of animal products often means fewer plants on the plate.

A diet heavy in burgers, cheese, and fried chicken leaves little room for spinach, beans, lentils, quinoa, or colorful vegetables — all of which provide magnesium, folate, antioxidants, and fiber. This imbalance means even people who "eat enough" can develop deficiencies.

4. Medications That Deplete Nutrients

One of the least-known contributors to deficiency is prescription medication. Common drugs silently rob the body of vitamins and minerals:

- **Proton pump inhibitors (acid blockers):** deplete magnesium, calcium, and B12.
- **Statins (cholesterol drugs):** reduce coenzyme Q10.
- **Diuretics:** wash out potassium and magnesium.
- **Oral contraceptives:** lower B vitamins, zinc, and magnesium.
- **Metformin (diabetes drug):** depletes B12 and folate.

Millions take these medications daily without being told they're also losing essential nutrients.

5. Lifestyle Factors

Modern living accelerates nutrient depletion. Chronic stress burns through magnesium and vitamin C. Alcohol drains B vitamins and zinc. Smoking depletes vitamin C. Lack of sunlight leads to vitamin D deficiency. Even something as common as excess caffeine can lower calcium and magnesium over time.

Deficiency isn't about eating less — it's about eating the wrong things while living in ways that burn through what little we do get.

How Deficiencies Lead to Disease

Nutrients aren't just "extras" to round out a balanced diet. They are the spark plugs of life. Every single biochemical reaction in the body requires vitamins, minerals, or enzymes as cofactors. Without enough of them, the system falters.

Think of the body as a factory. The macronutrients — carbs, proteins, and fats — are the raw materials. But without the right micronutrients, the machines can't run. Production slows, errors pile up, breakdowns happen, and eventually, the factory fails.

Here are just a few ways long-term deficiencies pave the road to disease:

- **Immune Breakdown:** Low vitamin C and zinc weaken the body's ability to fight infection. That's why deficient people catch every cold and take longer to recover.
- **Bone Fragility:** Low vitamin D and calcium silently weaken bones for decades before showing up as osteoporosis or fractures.
- **Cardiovascular Disease:** Low magnesium and potassium increase risk of high blood pressure and arrhythmias, while folate deficiency raises homocysteine, a marker linked to heart disease.
- **Diabetes:** Magnesium deficiency makes cells resistant to insulin, setting the stage for type 2 diabetes.
- **Cancer Risk:** Low antioxidants mean DNA damage goes unrepaired, mutations accumulate, and cancer risk rises.
- **Neurological Decline:** Low B12 and folate lead to nerve damage, memory problems, and higher dementia risk.
- **Mental Health:** Deficiencies in omega-3s, vitamin D, and B vitamins contribute to depression and anxiety.

Disease doesn't appear overnight. It grows in the cracks created by deficiency. A little fatigue here, a little insomnia there — until one day it's labeled "chronic illness."

This is why prevention matters. By the time deficiency shows up on a blood test or scan, the body has been compensating for years. The damage is already in motion. The only way forward is to stay nourished before symptoms appear.

The Plant-Based Solution

Here's the good news: deficiencies don't have to be your story. The solution isn't exotic powders, miracle pills, or expensive supplements. The answer has always been right in front of us: **plants.**

Whole, plant-based foods are the richest sources of nutrients on Earth. Fruits, vegetables, legumes, nuts, seeds, and whole grains deliver vitamins, minerals, antioxidants, and phytonutrients in the exact packages nature designed for human health.

Why Plants Work So Well

1. **Density:** Ounce for ounce, plants contain far more vitamins and minerals than meat, dairy, or processed foods. A cup of kale contains more calcium than a slice of cheese, without the saturated fat. A handful of pumpkin seeds delivers more magnesium than a steak.
2. **Synergy:** Nutrients in plants don't work in isolation — they cooperate. Vitamin C enhances iron absorption. Flavonoids protect vitamin E. Fiber feeds gut bacteria, which produce B vitamins. When you eat plants, you're not just getting nutrients, you're getting **networks of nutrients that activate each other.**
3. **Balance:** Supplements often deliver single nutrients in doses the body can't absorb properly. Whole plants deliver them in natural ratios the body recognizes and uses efficiently.
4. **Protection:** Phytonutrients — unique compounds like carotenoids, flavonoids, and polyphenols — act

as antioxidants, anti-inflammatories, and even natural detoxifiers. These compounds aren't found in animal foods, and they can't be replicated in a pill.

Eating the Rainbow

The simplest way to correct deficiencies is to eat colorfully. Each color signals unique compounds and nutrients:

- **Red foods (tomatoes, strawberries, red peppers):** rich in lycopene and vitamin C.
- **Orange foods (carrots, sweet potatoes, oranges):** high in beta-carotene, converted into vitamin A.
- **Yellow foods (bananas, corn, squash):** provide potassium and lutein.
- **Green foods (spinach, broccoli, kale):** packed with magnesium, folate, calcium, and vitamin K.
- **Blue/Purple foods (blueberries, grapes, eggplant):** anthocyanins for brain and heart health.
- **Brown/White foods (garlic, onions, mushrooms, oats):** allicin, selenium, and immune boosters.

When your plate looks like a rainbow, deficiencies don't stand a chance.

Stories That Make It Real

Stories bring theory to life. Here are a few that illustrate how powerful nutrient repletion can be:

- **Maria's Fatigue:** A 42-year-old mother of two felt exhausted every afternoon. Her doctor suggested antidepressants. A nutritionist checked her ferritin (iron stores) — it was low. After shifting to lentils, spinach, black beans, and fortified plant foods, Maria's energy soared. Her depression lifted without medication.

- **James and Restless Legs:** A 55-year-old mechanic suffered nightly restless legs that ruined his sleep. Instead of another sedative, he added magnesium-rich foods like pumpkin seeds, almonds, and Swiss chard. Within days, his legs calmed and his sleep improved.
- **Sophia's Anxiety:** A college student plagued by anxiety attacks learned her diet of pizza, ramen, and soda left her deficient in B vitamins and magnesium. With oatmeal, leafy greens, beans, and sunflower seeds, her panic attacks eased, and her concentration improved.
- **David's Heart Palpitations:** A businessman had irregular heartbeats. His cardiologist recommended beta blockers, but further tests showed low potassium and magnesium. He began eating bananas, sweet potatoes, beans, and leafy greens daily. The arrhythmias faded.

Each of these cases demonstrates the same truth: **the body wasn't broken, it was undernourished.**

Key Takeaways

- Nutrient deficiencies are common, even in wealthy countries.
- Deficiencies rarely look dramatic; they feel like fatigue, anxiety, poor sleep, or brain fog.
- Modern farming, processing, medications, and lifestyle choices strip nutrients from our bodies.

- Disease grows in the cracks left behind by long-term deficiencies.
- Plant-based foods naturally replenish what's missing — no pills required.

Expanded Action Steps

Changing nutrition doesn't have to be overwhelming. Small, consistent steps reverse deficiencies over time. Here's a practical starter plan:

1. **Add a color today.** If your plate is beige, add something green or red. One new color daily ensures variety.
2. **Swap one processed food.** Replace chips with almonds, soda with sparkling water, white rice with quinoa.
3. **Prioritize magnesium.** Add pumpkin seeds, spinach, or black beans at least once daily.
4. **Get natural vitamin D.** Spend 15 minutes in the sun, or include fortified plant milks if sunlight is scarce.
5. **Strengthen iron intake.** Combine beans or lentils with vitamin C–rich foods (like tomatoes or citrus) to maximize absorption.
6. **Balance B vitamins.** Enjoy whole grains, leafy greens, and legumes every day.
7. **Hydrate smart.** Water helps transport nutrients; aim for steady hydration.
8. **Know your medications.** If you take prescriptions, learn which nutrients they deplete and adjust your diet accordingly.

9. **Build consistency, not perfection.** Missing a day won't harm you; what matters is the trend.

Closing Message

Your body isn't falling apart. It's asking for fuel. Fatigue, mood swings, and aches aren't random — they're signals. Deficiencies are the body's cry for help. The answer isn't another pill. The answer is nourishment.

The truth is simple: **disease begins with deficiency — and health begins with abundance.**

In ***The P53 Diet & Lifestyle***, I explained how deficiencies open the door to disease by weakening immunity and destabilizing hormones. In my research on pharmaceuticals, I showed how common drugs quietly strip away vital nutrients. This book simplifies the message even further: deficiencies aren't rare. They're everywhere. And you can fix them.

Health is not about deprivation. It's about restoration. Every apple, every bowl of beans, every handful of seeds is medicine. Every color on your plate is a prescription. Every day you move closer to abundance, your body thanks you.

This is the first step of your journey: understanding that deficiencies are the silent epidemic — but also the easiest to heal. By choosing whole plant foods, you give your body exactly what it has been asking for all along.

Chapter 2

Germ Theory vs. Terrain Theory: Rethinking Health

When people get sick, most assume it's because of germs. A virus, a bacterium, or some invisible invader came in from the outside and made them ill. This way of thinking is so common it feels like common sense. Germs equal sickness — end of story.

This is called Germ Theory. It became popular in the late 1800s when scientists like Louis Pasteur showed that certain microbes were linked to certain diseases. It gave medicine an easy villain: germs are the problem, drugs and disinfectants are the solution.

But Germ Theory is a false picture.

There is another way of seeing health and disease. It's called **Terrain Theory.** Instead of focusing on what invades the body, it focuses on the state of the body itself. If your terrain — your immune system, nutrient status, gut health, stress resilience — is strong, germs rarely matter. If your terrain is weak, even mild exposures can bring you down.

This is a crucial shift in perspective. Germs are everywhere, all the time. They always have been and always will be. But whether or not you get sick depends far more on the soil (your terrain) than on the seed (the germ).

Pasteur himself, the father of Germ Theory, is said to have admitted later in life: ***"The microbe is nothing; the terrain is everything."*** Whether or not he phrased it exactly that way, the evidence is clear: two people can encounter the same germ, yet one thrives while the other suffers. The deciding factor isn't the germ. It's the terrain.

Germ Theory: A Narrow Lens

Germ Theory created a narrow way of thinking: germs are the enemy, and health is about constant defense. Sanitize the hands. Spray the surfaces. Take the pill. Kill the invader.

That mindset misses the bigger truth: germs don't act alone. They are opportunists. They take advantage when the body is weak, depleted, or stressed.

If Germ Theory were the whole story, everyone exposed to the same germ would get sick in the same way. But that's not reality.

- In a family of five, one person gets a stomach bug, two feel fine, and the others barely notice.
- In a classroom, half the kids catch a cold while the other half sail through.
- In workplaces, some employees are constantly run down while others hardly ever take a sick day.

If germs alone dictated outcomes, these differences wouldn't exist. The missing variable is the terrain.

Terrain Theory: A Deeper Understanding

Terrain Theory says the key question is not *"**Which germ caused this?**"* but *"**What weakened the body enough to let this happen?**"*

Instead of putting the spotlight on the invader, Terrain Theory shines it on the host. And the truth is, most of the modern factors that erode health come from inside our daily lives, not from outside attackers.

- **Diet:** A menu of processed food, sugar, and oils robs the body of the vitamins and minerals that immunity depends on.
- **Sleep:** Without deep rest, the immune system can't recover or defend.
- **Stress:** Chronic tension floods the body with cortisol, which weakens immune response.
- **Toxins:** Alcohol, smoking, pollution, pesticides, and household chemicals all place extra burden on the body.
- **Deficiencies:** Low vitamin D, magnesium, zinc, or B vitamins leave the immune system without its tools.

When the terrain is weak, even mild exposures create illness. When the terrain is strong, the same exposures bounce off with little or no effect.

This is not fringe theory — it is how human biology works. Your body is an ecosystem, and just like a garden, it thrives or fails depending on the soil.

Everyday Proof

Terrain Theory isn't abstract. You see it every day if you pay attention:

- **Colds:** Some people catch every sniffle; others rarely get sick. The difference isn't the germ — it's the terrain.
- **Food poisoning:** A group eats the same meal. One ends up in the ER, others just feel a bit off, and some feel nothing at all. Same bacteria, different terrain.
- **Childhood illnesses:** In a group of kids, one constantly battles ear infections while another seems immune. Same environment, different terrain.
- **The workplace effect:** One employee burns through sick days every year, while another rarely misses a shift. The difference is resilience, not exposure.

The germ is like a spark.
The terrain is like the forest floor.
Dry brush ignites quickly. Healthy, damp soil resists the flame.

Why Terrain Matters More Today

In the 1800s, it made sense to fixate on germs. Cities were filthy, sanitation was poor, and people were dying of infections from contaminated water and unwashed hands. In that world, identifying microbes was a breakthrough.

But today, those conditions are no longer the primary threat. We live in a different health crisis. Modern epidemics are chronic diseases — heart disease, diabetes, cancer, autoimmune conditions, dementia. None of these are caused by a single germ. They are caused by **weak terrain.**

And yet, most of modern medicine still thinks like it's stuck in the 19th century: identify the "enemy," kill it, and suppress the symptoms. That may work for emergencies, but it does nothing to restore resilience.

- Processed food keeps the body inflamed.
- Sedentary lifestyles weaken circulation and immunity.
- Stress and sleeplessness wear down defenses.
- Chemicals and pollutants overload the system.

Terrain Theory doesn't reject Germ Theory. It simply shows us the larger picture. Germs exist, but they only thrive when the soil is right. Instead of fighting endless battles against microbes, the wiser approach is to strengthen the terrain so they rarely matter.

The Science of Terrain

If Terrain Theory sounds like common sense — strengthen the body, and you resist illness — it's because it is. But it's also backed by science, far more than most people realize. Modern immunology, microbiology, and nutrition research all confirm one central truth: **your inner environment matters more than the outer invader.**

Let's explore the science that makes Terrain Theory real.

The Immune System: Your Living Defense

Your immune system is not a wall that either keeps germs out or lets them in. It's a living, dynamic army that depends on nutrients, rest, and balance.

- **White blood cells** patrol like security guards, constantly scanning for invaders. But without zinc and vitamin C, their radios don't work, and they can't communicate.
- **T-cells and B-cells** are the specialists, learning to recognize threats and build long-term defenses. Without vitamin D, they can't activate properly.

- **Natural killer cells** are like the body's SWAT team, eliminating dangerous cells before they spread. Without magnesium, their energy systems fail.
- **Antioxidants** like glutathione, vitamin E, and carotenoids are the shields, preventing damage from free radicals. Without them, DNA and proteins become vulnerable.

In other words, immunity is terrain-dependent. A germ may arrive, but whether it gains ground depends entirely on whether the defense system is nourished and ready.

The Microbiome: The Terrain Within

Perhaps the most powerful scientific validation of Terrain Theory comes from the human microbiome — the trillions of microbes living in your gut, skin, lungs, and everywhere else.

For decades, Germ Theory cast microbes as the enemy. But the microbiome has flipped that view on its head. Most microbes are not only harmless but essential for health.

- Gut bacteria produce B vitamins and vitamin K.
- They train and balance the immune system, preventing overreaction.
- They protect against pathogens by competing for space and resources.
- They influence mood by producing serotonin and dopamine precursors.

When the terrain of the microbiome is healthy — diverse, plant-fed, fiber-rich — germs have a hard time taking over. But when the terrain is weak — starved of fiber, overloaded with sugar and antibiotics — harmful bacteria dominate, setting the stage for illness.

Science now confirms what Terrain Theory has said for centuries: **it's not the presence of microbes that matters, it's the balance of the terrain they live in.**

Nutrient Pathways: Fuel for Defense

Every biochemical pathway that protects your body depends on nutrients:

- **Iron and copper** allow red blood cells to carry oxygen.
- **Magnesium** powers over 300 enzymatic reactions, from muscle function to DNA repair.
- **Zinc** enables over 100 enzymes, many of them immune-related.
- **B vitamins** drive energy metabolism and nerve function.
- **Vitamin C** rebuilds collagen, heals tissues, and neutralizes free radicals.

Take any of these away, and the defense system weakens. The germ may be the trigger, but the deficiency is the reason it takes hold.

This is why two people exposed to the same bacteria have different outcomes. One has a nutrient-rich terrain, so the immune system neutralizes the invader. The other has gaps, so the invader spreads.

Epigenetics: Terrain Shapes Expression

One of the most exciting areas of science is **epigenetics** — how lifestyle and environment switch genes on and off. You are not just a victim of your DNA. Genes load the gun, but environment pulls the trigger.

What determines whether "bad" genes express themselves? The terrain.

- Nutrient sufficiency can silence harmful genetic expressions.
- Antioxidants protect DNA from mutations.
- Stress and toxins can flip genes in the wrong direction.
- Exercise, sleep, and plant-based foods promote gene repair.

This means terrain doesn't just affect day-to-day immunity. It shapes your long-term destiny. Chronic diseases like cancer, heart disease, and even dementia are not dictated by germs — they emerge from decades of weakened terrain.

Chronic Diseases: Proof of Weak Terrain

Think about the leading killers of today:

- **Heart disease** comes from inflammation, clogged arteries, and nutrient imbalances — not from germs.
- **Diabetes** comes from insulin resistance, magnesium deficiency, and processed food diets — not from germs.
- **Cancer** emerges when oxidative stress and DNA damage overwhelm repair systems — not from germs.
- **Autoimmune conditions** develop when the immune system misfires due to gut imbalance and deficiencies — not from germs.
- **Dementia** grows from years of oxidative stress, vascular decline, and nutrient shortages — not from germs.

If Germ Theory explained everything, drugs that kill germs would solve these problems. But they don't. Because these conditions are about terrain, not invaders.

The Terrain Analogy: Garden or Garbage Heap

Think of your body as a garden.

If the soil is rich, watered, and full of nutrients, healthy plants flourish, and weeds struggle to survive. That's strong terrain.

But if the soil is depleted, dry, and filled with trash, weeds take over. That's weak terrain.

Germs are like weed seeds. They're everywhere, carried on the wind, impossible to avoid. But whether they sprout depends entirely on the soil. Blame the seed if you want, but the real solution is to tend the garden.

Why Science Overwhelmingly Supports Terrain

You may not hear about Terrain Theory in everyday health advice, but modern science overwhelmingly confirms it:

- Studies show vitamin D deficiency correlates with higher rates of respiratory illness.
- Zinc supplementation reduces the length and severity of colds.
- Magnesium deficiency is linked to increased risk of diabetes, hypertension, and depression.
- Fiber-rich diets support gut bacteria that suppress harmful pathogens.
- Antioxidant intake reduces markers of DNA damage and inflammation.

Every one of these findings points back to the same truth: **germs don't determine health — terrain does.**

Building Strong Terrain

If terrain is what determines whether disease takes root, then the real question becomes: **how do we strengthen it?**

Unlike Germ Theory, which focuses on fighting invaders, Terrain Theory empowers you to focus on what you can control every day. Germs are everywhere. They always will be. But your terrain is in your hands.

The pillars of terrain health are simple, timeless, and free:

1. Nutrition: Fueling the Terrain

The terrain runs on nutrients. Without them, the immune system has no ammunition. With them, the body becomes a fortress.

- **Fruits and Vegetables:** These are the frontline. Rich in vitamin C, carotenoids, flavonoids, and minerals, they provide the antioxidants and co-factors your cells need.
- **Legumes and Whole Grains:** Beans, lentils, oats, and quinoa stabilize blood sugar, fuel gut bacteria, and provide magnesium, folate, and zinc.
- **Nuts and Seeds:** Almonds, walnuts, flaxseeds, chia, and pumpkin seeds supply essential fatty acids, vitamin E, and minerals like selenium.
- **Herbs and Spices:** Garlic, turmeric, ginger, and oregano are natural antimicrobials that support the immune system without harming beneficial microbes.

Eating a rainbow every day isn't just a slogan — it's the most powerful terrain medicine we know.

2. Restorative Sleep

Sleep is when the terrain repairs itself. White blood cells reset, hormones rebalance, tissues heal. Just one night of poor sleep reduces natural killer cell activity by nearly 50%. Chronic sleep deprivation leaves the terrain wide open to invaders.

Building your terrain means protecting sleep: 7–9 hours of deep, consistent rest. Dark room. Cool temperature. No screens before bed. Treat sleep as seriously as you treat food.

3. Movement

Exercise isn't about burning calories. It's about strengthening terrain. Movement increases circulation, delivering nutrients to tissues and removing waste. It enhances lymphatic flow, which is how immune cells travel. It reduces chronic inflammation and builds resilience.

You don't need extreme workouts. Walking, gardening, stretching, cycling, dancing — all count. Consistency is more powerful than intensity.

4. Stress Management

Chronic stress floods the body with cortisol, which weakens immune function and depletes nutrients. Short bursts of stress are natural. Constant stress erodes terrain.

Daily practices like meditation, prayer, deep breathing, journaling, or time in nature restore balance. Even five minutes of stillness lowers stress hormones and strengthens immunity.

5. Toxin Reduction

Every toxin the body processes — from alcohol to pesticides to cleaning chemicals — diverts resources away from immunity. The more toxins, the weaker the terrain.

Simple steps strengthen the terrain:

- Limit alcohol.
- Quit smoking.
- Choose organic or wash produce thoroughly.
- Use natural cleaning products.
- Stay hydrated to flush waste.

Terrain health thrives in a clean environment, inside and out.

Stories That Make It Real

Sometimes the science feels abstract until you see it in real lives. Here are a few stories that bring Terrain Theory to life:

- **Carla the Teacher:** Every winter, Carla caught three or four colds. She blamed the kids in her classroom for "spreading germs." But when she began eating more vegetables, cutting back on sugar, and going to bed earlier, something changed: she went an entire winter without getting sick. The children hadn't changed — her terrain had.
- **Mark the Traveler:** Mark was a consultant who flew constantly for work. Every trip seemed to end with stomach trouble or respiratory infections. When he began eating fermented foods, taking fiber seriously, and drinking more water, his gut terrain strengthened. The "travel bugs" stopped being a problem.
- **Angela and Anxiety:** Angela struggled with both anxiety and constant sinus infections. Instead of an-

other prescription, she tried focusing on terrain: daily walks, meditation, and magnesium-rich foods. Her anxiety eased, her sleep improved, and the sinus infections faded. The germs didn't disappear — but her resilience did the work.

Key Takeaways

- Germs are everywhere, but whether they cause illness depends on terrain.
- Terrain Theory is supported by science: immunity, microbiome, nutrient pathways, and epigenetics all confirm it.
- Chronic diseases prove the terrain principle — they don't come from germs, they come from long-term weakness.
- Building terrain is simple: nutrition, sleep, movement, stress reduction, and toxin avoidance.

Action Steps

To make Terrain Theory practical, here are steps you can start today:

1. **Eat the Rainbow:** Add at least three colors of fruits or vegetables to every meal.
2. **Protect Sleep:** Aim for 7–9 hours with a consistent bedtime.
3. **Move Daily:** Walk for 30 minutes, stretch, or do any joyful activity.
4. **Calm Stress:** Take five minutes daily for deep breathing or quiet reflection.

5. **Cut Toxins:** Swap one processed snack for whole food, or replace a harsh cleaner with a natural option.
6. **Support the Gut:** Add fiber, beans, or fermented foods daily to nourish your microbiome.
7. **Hydrate:** Drink water steadily throughout the day to keep terrain flushed and strong.

Over time, these small actions create terrain that is resilient, balanced, and difficult for illness to penetrate.

Closing Message

Germs will always be here. You can't control them. You can't sanitize them away. But you can control your terrain.

The truth is simple: **don't fear the spark — strengthen the ground it falls on.**

In *The P53 Diet & Lifestyle*, I explained how strong immune systems depend more on nutrient density than on fighting germs. In my cancer research, I showed how weak terrain allows abnormal cells to grow like weeds in depleted soil.

This book keeps the message simple: stop fearing germs. Start strengthening your terrain. Every choice you make — every plate of food, every hour of sleep, every moment of calm, every walk outside — is a way of tending the soil of your body. Strong terrain doesn't just fight illness. It prevents it. It creates health from the inside out.

Chapter 3

Animal Products: Meat, Dairy, Eggs, & Seafood

For decades, animal products have been marketed as the foundation of strength and health.

- Meat builds muscle.
- Milk builds bones.
- Eggs are "nature's perfect protein."
- Seafood is "heart-healthy."
- Honey is "nature's sugar."

These slogans have been repeated so often they feel like cultural truths. Entire industries built fortunes on them. But when you peel back the glossy marketing, the shine fades quickly.

Behind the promises are cholesterol, hormones, antibiotics, heavy metals, and toxins that don't build health — they erode it.

The truth is simple: **animal foods are not necessary for survival. In fact, they often do more harm than good.**

Meat: The Protein Myth

Meat is praised as the ultimate protein source, the building block of strength. But protein wrapped in animal flesh carries dangerous baggage:

- **Cholesterol & Saturated Fat** – clog arteries and drive heart disease.
- **IGF-1 Stimulation** – accelerates cell growth, including cancer cells.
- **Heme Iron** – absorbed without regulation, building up and creating oxidative stress, DNA damage, and increased cancer risk.
- **Cooking By-Products** – high-heat cooking forms carcinogenic compounds (HCAs and AGEs).

People think they're eating strength. In reality, they're eating weakness dressed as strength.

Iron: Why Source Matters

Iron is essential for life — it carries oxygen in blood and powers enzymes. But not all iron behaves the same:

- **Non-Heme Iron (plants):** Absorbed with regulation. Your body takes what it needs and leaves the rest.
- **Heme Iron (animals):** Forces its way into cells whether you need it or not. This "unregulated entry" leads to oxidative stress, DNA damage, and cancer-causing compounds.

Studies consistently show high heme iron intake is linked to colon, breast, and prostate cancers — while plant iron shows no such risk.

People eat meat for "healthy iron," but the form they get often fuels the very diseases they fear.

Dairy: The Calcium Lie

Milk has long been sold as bone protection. Yet paradoxically, countries with the highest dairy intake also suffer the highest osteoporosis rates.

Why?

- Dairy delivers calcium, but also an acidic load that forces the body to pull calcium from bones.
- Dairy contains hormones and growth factors linked to cancer.
- Lactose intolerance affects most of the world, causing bloating and digestive pain.

Instead of building bone, dairy contributes to fragility. The marketing promised strength. Biology delivers the opposite.

Casein and BCM-7: The Hidden Drug Effect

Cow's milk protein differs from human milk protein by just two amino acids. That tiny change produces a powerful effect.

When digested, bovine casein releases **BCM-7 (beta-casomorphin-7)**, a peptide that acts like an opioid:

- It binds to opioid receptors in the brain.
- It alters mood and pain response.
- It may slow digestion and worsen inflammation.

This explains why cheese feels addictive. People say they "can't give it up." That's not weakness — that's chemistry. BCM-7 is acting on the brain like a drug.

Human breast milk, by contrast, produces peptides that support immune and brain development without the opioid effect. Cow's milk was made for calves, not humans.

Eggs: Nature's "Perfect" Deception

Eggs are marketed as "incredible, edible, perfect protein." But the reality is darker:

- **Cholesterol Bombs** – A single egg contains ~200 mg cholesterol, raising LDL ("bad") cholesterol and heart risk.
- **Diabetes Risk** – Studies link egg consumption to higher rates of type 2 diabetes.
- **Choline and TMAO** – Eggs are high in choline, which gut bacteria convert into TMAO (trimethylamine N-oxide), a compound strongly linked to artery damage and atherosclerosis.

So eggs deliver protein, yes — but at the cost of clogged arteries, higher heart risk, and harmful by-products. "Perfect" is the marketing, not the biology.

Seafood: Omega-3s with a Side of Toxins

Seafood is often praised as "heart healthy" because of omega-3 fatty acids. But the modern ocean tells a different story:

- **Mercury** – a neurotoxin that damages the brain and nerves.

- **PCBs & Dioxins** – industrial pollutants that cause cancer.
- **Microplastics** – now found in nearly all fish.

Yes, fish contain omega-3s — but you can get the same fats from flax, chia, hemp, walnuts, and algae, without the toxins.

The ocean is no longer clean. Fish have become chemical sponges.

Honey: Nature's Sugar, Still Sugar

Honey wears the halo of "natural," but your body processes it like any other sugar:

- Spikes blood sugar.
- Fuels inflammation.
- Contributes to weight gain and insulin resistance.

Yes, honey contains trace antioxidants, but fruit contains far more — along with fiber and hydration. Honey is not medicine. It's sugar with better PR.

If you want sweetness, eat fruit.

The Common Thread

Step back, and the pattern is clear:

- **Meat** fuels cancer and heart disease through heme iron, cholesterol, and IGF-1.
- **Dairy** disrupts hormones, weakens bones, and creates addictive peptides.
- **Eggs** deliver cholesterol and harmful by-products like TMAO.
- **Seafood** contains omega-3s laced with mercury, dioxins, and plastics.

· **Honey** is sugar in disguise.

Each contains something useful (protein, calcium, iron, omega-3s, sweetness), but each comes with baggage that plants simply don't carry.

Stories That Make It Real
Michael's Red Meat Wake-Up Call

Michael ate "lean" red meat daily. At 52, a colonoscopy revealed precancerous polyps. When he replaced meat with beans and grains, his cholesterol dropped, digestion improved, and his cancer risk fell.

Sandra's "Calcium" Mistake

Sandra drank milk daily for her bones, yet developed osteoporosis. Switching to greens, beans, and fortified plant milks stabilized her bone density.

Derek and the Cheese Craving

Derek couldn't quit cheese. When he finally cut it, his brain fog cleared and digestion improved. Later, he learned about BCM-7 — the addictive opioid peptide.

Linda's Egg Dilemma

Linda loved eggs for breakfast until her cholesterol hit 260. After cutting eggs, her cholesterol normalized and she was able to ditch statins.

Carlos and the Seafood Trap

Carlos ate salmon for his heart — until mercury toxicity caused numbness. When he switched to plant-based omega-3s, symptoms disappeared.

Key Takeaways

· Meat provides protein, but also heme iron and carcinogenic by-products.

- Dairy provides calcium, but also hormones, acid load, and BCM-7.
- Eggs provide protein, but also cholesterol and TMAO.
- Seafood provides omega-3s, but also heavy metals and plastics.
- Honey is sugar in disguise.

Plants provide the same nutrients — protein, calcium, iron, omega-3s, sweetness — without the baggage.

Action Steps

1. **Swap Protein** – Replace meat with beans, lentils, or tempeh.
2. **Strengthen Bones Naturally** – Use greens, beans, nuts, and fortified plant milks instead of dairy.
3. **Cut Eggs** – Try oatmeal, fruit, or chickpea scrambles instead.
4. **Go Fish-Free** – Get omega-3s from flax, chia, walnuts, or algae oil.
5. **Skip Honey** – Use dates, bananas, or applesauce for natural sweetness.

Closing Message

Animal foods have long been marketed as health builders. But when you strip away the illusion, they emerge as health destroyers.

The truth is simple: **plants give you everything you need — without the baggage that kills.**

Chapter 4

Fats & Oils: Sorting the Healthy from the Harmful

For decades, fat has been one of the most confusing subjects in nutrition.

- In the 1980s, fat was demonized. "Low-fat" everything lined supermarket shelves — cookies, yogurts, crackers. People believed fat itself was the villain behind obesity and heart disease.
- In the 2000s, fat was glorified. Atkins, paleo, and keto diets preached that carbs were the enemy and fat was salvation. Suddenly butter in coffee was "health food."
- Today, people are more confused than ever. Should you eat butter or avoid it? Is olive oil medicine or just calories? Is coconut oil superfood or saturated fat?

The truth is simpler than the marketing wars: **your body does need fat — but it needs the right kind, in the right form, and in the right amount.**

Fat is essential for cell membranes, brain function, hormone production, and nutrient absorption. But the source of the fat makes the difference between health and disease.

The Bad Fats
1. Trans Fats: Manufactured Poisons

Trans fats are artificial fats created by hydrogenating vegetable oils to make them solid at room temperature. They're found in margarine, shortening, fried foods, and processed snacks.

- They raise LDL cholesterol (bad).
- They lower HDL cholesterol (good).
- They inflame blood vessels.
- They increase risk of heart disease, diabetes, and dementia.

There is no safe level of trans fats. Many countries have banned them, but they still lurk in processed foods under labels like "partially hydrogenated oil."

2. Excess Saturated Fats: Artery Stiffeners

Saturated fats are found mainly in meat, cheese, butter, and coconut oil. The body can process them, but in modern diets, saturated fat intake is far beyond healthy levels.

- They raise total and LDL cholesterol.
- They stiffen arteries, impairing circulation.
- They promote insulin resistance.
- They fuel chronic inflammation.

Countries with high saturated fat consumption have some of the highest heart disease rates. Yet food marketing continues to push butter, cheese, and "grass-fed" beef as healthy indulgences. The baggage outweighs the benefits.

3. Refined Oils: The Industrial Product

Here's where most people get fooled. Bottles of corn oil, soybean oil, canola oil, and "vegetable oil" look harmless on the shelf. But these are not natural foods — they are industrial extracts.

To get oil out of a seed, chemical companies use hexane, a toxic solvent derived from petroleum. The process looks nothing like food preparation. Seeds are:

1. Ground into meal.
2. Washed in hexane to dissolve the oils.
3. Heated at high temperatures to remove the solvent.
4. Bleached and deodorized to hide the rancid smell.

By the end, the oil is stripped of fiber, protein, and most nutrients — leaving behind pure, oxidized fat molecules. Traces of hexane can remain, and while regulators call the levels "safe," the idea that your salad dressing was once bathed in a neurotoxic gasoline by-product is sobering.

These oils are unstable. They oxidize easily, especially when heated, producing aldehydes and free radicals that damage DNA and proteins. Studies link high refined oil intake to inflammation, heart disease, and obesity.

The Good Fats

Not all fats are the enemy. The body thrives on fats that come packaged in whole foods:

1. Omega-3s: The Inflammation Fighters

Omega-3 fatty acids reduce inflammation, lower triglycerides, improve brain function, and protect the heart. Best plant sources: flax, chia, hemp, walnuts, and algae.

2. Monounsaturated Fats: The Balancers

Found in olives, avocados, and almonds, these fats support healthy cholesterol levels, improve insulin sensitivity, and nourish the brain.

3. Whole-Food Fats: Nature's Packaging

Nuts, seeds, avocados, and whole olives provide fat wrapped in fiber, minerals, and antioxidants. This natural package slows absorption, prevents overconsumption, and adds protective compounds missing from oils.

Whole-food fats don't just give calories. They give balance.

The Hidden Dangers of Oil Processing

Oils may look pure and golden in a bottle, but the process that gets them there is anything but natural. To understand why refined oils are harmful, you need to see how they're made.

Step 1: The Seed is Stripped

Corn, soybeans, cottonseeds, rapeseeds (canola), and sunflowers aren't naturally oily to the touch. To get oil, the seeds must be:

- Cleaned, cracked, and ground into meal.
- Heated to high temperatures to release oil.

Already, many nutrients — vitamin E, phytosterols, carotenoids — are destroyed.

Step 2: Bathing in Hexane

The ground seeds are then washed with hexane, a petroleum-derived solvent. Hexane dissolves the oil molecules so they can be separated from the seed meal.

Hexane is classified as a neurotoxin. Inhaling it damages nerves and lungs. Workers must be protected when handling it. And while most of it is later evaporated out of the oil, trace amounts remain. Regulators allow it, claiming the levels are "safe." But does anyone really want solvent residue in their salad dressing?

Step 3: High-Heat Refining

The oil is then boiled to evaporate the hexane. This heating oxidizes delicate fatty acids, creating unstable compounds.

Step 4: Bleaching and Deodorizing

The oil turns rancid in the process, so it must be bleached to remove color and deodorized to remove the smell. The final product looks clean, but it is **chemically altered, nutrient-depleted, and oxidized.**

What began as a whole food (a seed) has become an industrial chemical extract.

And this is what most people use daily for frying, sautéing, baking, and even in so-called "health foods."

Oils and Oxidation

The biggest problem with refined oils is not just the processing, but what happens next: **oxidation.**

Polyunsaturated oils like soybean, corn, and canola are unstable. When exposed to air, light, or heat, their fatty acids break apart, forming aldehydes, peroxides, and free radicals. These compounds:

- Damage cell membranes.
- Mutate DNA.

- Trigger chronic inflammation.
- Age tissues prematurely.

Every time oil smokes in your pan, you're creating these compounds — and then eating them.

Fat Metabolism: More Than Calories

We often think of fat simply as a "dense calorie source" (9 calories per gram). But fat is more than fuel — it is also convertible currency inside the body.

Fat → Fatty Acids + Glycerol

When fat (triglycerides) is broken down, it releases:

- **Fatty acids** → burned for energy or stored.
- **Glycerol backbone** → a simple sugar alcohol.

Glycerol → Glucose

The glycerol backbone is converted in the liver via gluconeogenesis into glucose.

This means: **excess dietary fat can ultimately be turned into sugar inside your body.**

Why This Matters for Cancer

Cancer cells thrive on glucose. They are metabolically abnormal, preferring to ferment glucose into lactate (the "Warburg effect") even when oxygen is available. This gives them a constant appetite for sugar.

Most people think sugar only comes from carbs. But here's the hidden truth: **excess fats also end up feeding cancer cells.**

- Triglycerides break down into glycerol.
- Glycerol is turned into glucose in the liver.

· That glucose enters the bloodstream.
· Cancer cells absorb it greedily through GLUT trans-
porters.

In other words:

· Sugar feeds cancer.
· Refined carbs feed cancer.
· But so do **oils and excess fats**, once they are con-
verted into glucose.

This is why high-fat diets, especially when combined with refined oils, can accelerate cancer growth. They not only inflame
the body but also provide hidden glucose for tumors.

Fats, Hormones, and Inflammation

Excess fats do more than fuel cancer. They also:

· **Inflame tissues:** Omega-6–heavy oils (corn, soybean, sunflower) are precursors to arachidonic acid,
which promotes pro-inflammatory prostaglandins.
· **Alter hormones:** Saturated fats increase estrogen
and testosterone levels, both linked to hormone-driven cancers (breast, prostate).
· **Block insulin sensitivity:** High fat impairs glucose
transport, leading to higher blood sugar — again feeding cancer cells indirectly.

This creates a perfect storm: more inflammation, more hormone stimulation, more glucose — the terrain where cancer
thrives.

Oils vs. Whole-Food Fats

It's important to separate refined oils from whole-food fats.

- A walnut contains fat, yes, but it also contains fiber, magnesium, selenium, and antioxidants that protect against oxidation.
- Flaxseeds provide omega-3s packaged with lignans — compounds that block hormone-driven cancer.
- Avocado provides fat alongside potassium and carotenoids.

These foods deliver fat in balance with protective compounds. Oils strip that protection away. What's left is a calorie bomb that oxidizes easily, fuels inflammation, and — through glycerol — helps feed the very diseases people are trying to avoid.

Stories That Make It Real
Tony's Olive Oil Trap

Tony thought he was eating the "healthy Mediterranean diet." He poured olive oil over his salads, dipped bread in it, and sautéed every dish with it. But his weight refused to budge. His cholesterol crept higher. When he learned that olive oil was just liquid fat with 120 calories per tablespoon, he swapped it for whole olives, and avocado. Within months, the pounds began melting away, his cholesterol dropped, and his energy returned. The problem wasn't fat — it was *oil*.

Maria's Fried Food Pain

Maria, a 48-year-old nurse, suffered with aching joints. She assumed it was age. But her diet was heavy in fried foods: French fries, fried chicken, chips. When she cut out fried oils and switched to baked potatoes, roasted vegetables, and raw nuts, the difference was dramatic. Within weeks, her joint inflammation eased, her hands no longer swelled, and her mobility returned. Removing oxidized oils was like removing fuel from a fire.

Jared and the "Healthy Keto" Myth

Jared tried a keto diet, believing fat was harmless as long as carbs were low. He lived on butter coffee, bacon, and cheese. At first, he lost weight. But soon his blood sugar spiked, his triglycerides soared, and a scan revealed fatty liver. He learned why: excess fat can be converted to glucose via glycerol, which fed his blood sugar and inflamed his liver. Once he dropped oils and animal fats and added beans, fruits, and greens, his labs normalized. The illusion of "fat as savior" had nearly wrecked him.

Anita's Cancer Recovery Support

Anita was undergoing treatment for breast cancer. Her oncologist warned her to avoid sugar, but no one mentioned oils. When she read about how glycerol from fat can be converted to glucose — and how cancer cells thrive on glucose — she decided to cut out oils, butter, and fried foods. She focused on whole grains, beans, vegetables, fruits, and seeds. Her doctors were amazed at how stable her bloodwork remained during treatment. Oils were out, but nourishment was in.

These stories point to the same lesson: **fats matter, but the form and source matter more.**

Key Takeaways

- **Bad fats:**
  - **Trans fats** are poisons with no safe level.

- **Saturated fats** (meat, butter, cheese, coconut oil) stiffen arteries and fuel disease.
- **Refined oils** are industrial extracts made with hexane, stripped of nutrients, and prone to oxidation.
- **Hidden cancer connection:**
  - Fat breaks down into fatty acids + glycerol.
  - Glycerol is converted into glucose.
  - Glucose feeds cancer cells.
- **Good fats:**
  - **Omega-3s** (flax, chia, hemp, walnuts, algae) fight inflammation and protect the brain.
  - **Monounsaturated fats** (olives, avocados, almonds) support healthy cholesterol balance.
  - **Whole-food fats** come packaged with fiber, minerals, and antioxidants that oils lack.
- **Cooking oils are calorie bombs:** 120 calories per tablespoon with no fiber, no protection, and high oxidation risk when heated.

Action Steps

Here's how to begin transitioning away from harmful fats and oils:

1. **Ditch the Bottle**
   - Stop buying bottles of corn, soybean, canola, or "vegetable oil."
   - Replace with whole-food fats like avocado, nuts, and seeds.
2. **Change How You Cook**
   - Instead of frying or sautéing in oil, try water sauté, broth cooking, or dry roasting.

· Use parchment paper or silicone mats to bake without oil.

3. **Rethink Salad Dressing**
   · Blend avocado, mango, or lemon for creamy dressings.
   · Try balsamic vinegar with herbs instead of oil.

4. **Add Daily Omega-3s**
   · 1 tablespoon of ground flaxseed or chia seed daily supports brain and heart health.

5. **Watch Out for Hidden Oils**
   · Read labels on breads, crackers, and snacks. Many contain soybean or palm oil.
   · Choose minimally processed foods with no added oils.

6. **Track Inflammation**
   · Pay attention to how your joints, digestion, and skin respond when oils are cut out. Most people notice improvement within weeks.

Closing Message

Fat has been misunderstood for decades. It isn't the villain or the hero — it's the source that matters.

· **Refined oils** are industrial products, often extracted with toxic hexane, stripped of nutrients, and oxidized into harmful compounds.
· **Animal fats** are loaded with cholesterol and saturated fat that fuel heart disease, diabetes, and cancer.
· **Excess fats**, whether from butter, oil, or fried food, break down into glucose that can feed cancer cells — the very opposite of healing.

But whole-food fats — nuts, seeds, avocados, olives — are protective. They deliver fat in nature's package, alongside antioxidants, minerals, and fiber. They satisfy, nourish, and heal.

In **The P53 Diet & Lifestyle**, I showed how oils drive chronic disease and how plant fats heal. This book simplifies it: **don't fear fat — fear oils and animal fat. Whole-food plant fats heal.**

When you choose whole foods instead of bottles of oil or chunks of butter, you shift the balance of your terrain. You remove the toxins, calm the inflammation, and deny cancer its hidden fuel.

The truth is simple: **every meal is a chance to heal or to harm. Choose the fats that heal.**

Chapter 5

Sugar & Carbohydrates: Sweet Lies and Real Energy

Ask ten people about carbs and sugar, and you'll get ten different answers:

- "Carbs make you fat."
- "Sugar causes diabetes."
- "You need carbs for energy."
- "All carbs are the same."

No wonder everyone is confused. For decades, diet wars have painted carbohydrates as villains, miracle foods, or both. Low-carb, high-carb, keto, paleo, Atkins, Zone — each one claimed the truth.

But here's the reality: **not all carbs are created equal.** Some heal. Some harm. Knowing the difference is the key to health.

Carbohydrates 101

Carbohydrates are your body's primary energy source. Every cell runs on glucose — your muscles, your brain, your organs, your immune system. Even your red blood cells and certain brain cells can **only** use glucose for fuel.

But not all carbohydrates are the same:

- **Complex Carbohydrates** → found in whole foods like fruit, beans, vegetables, and whole grains. They come wrapped in fiber, water, vitamins, minerals, and antioxidants. They digest slowly, giving steady energy and nourishment.
- **Simple Refined Carbohydrates** → found in soda, candy, white bread, pastries, and processed foods. Stripped of fiber and nutrients, they flood the bloodstream, spike blood sugar, crash energy, and fuel disease.

One group builds life. The other drains it.

The Sugar Trap

The biggest culprit in modern diets is refined sugar. It hides everywhere:

- Ketchup, barbecue sauce, salad dressings.
- Protein bars and "energy" drinks.
- Breakfast cereals and flavored yogurts.
- Bread, crackers, even canned soups.

The average person consumes over 150 pounds of sugar per year, much of it hidden. This overload does more than add empty calories — it destabilizes the terrain of the body.

Sugar excess drives:

- **Insulin resistance → diabetes.** Constant sugar spikes force insulin to work overtime until cells stop responding.
- **Chronic inflammation → heart disease.** Sugar promotes oxidative stress and vascular damage.
- **Weight gain → obesity.** Extra sugar is converted into fat and stored in the liver and belly.
- **Fuel for cancer → tumor growth.** Cancer cells are sugar addicts. They thrive on glucose.

In **Taste Versus Cancer**, I explained how sugar creates the perfect terrain for tumors. Starve cancer of sugar, and its growth slows. Flood it with sugar, and it spreads like wildfire.

The Carb Confusion

Here's the great irony: while refined sugar is deadly, real carbohydrates are healing.

Look at the longest-lived populations on earth:

- **Okinawans (Japan):** 70% of their calories came from sweet potatoes, plus rice, beans, and vegetables.
- **Sardinians (Italy):** Beans, lentils, barley, and sourdough bread formed the bulk of their diet.
- **Nicoyans (Costa Rica):** Corn, beans, and squash — the "three sisters" — formed their nutritional base.
- **Tarahumara (Mexico):** Famous for endurance running, their diet was 80% corn, beans, and squash.

Carbs made up **60–80% of their calories.** And the results? Low obesity, almost no diabetes, rare heart disease, and long lifespans.

Compare that to modern low-carb, high-meat societies — plagued with obesity, cancer, and cardiovascular disease. The difference is not carbs themselves. It's the source of the carbs.

Why Whole-Food Carbs Heal

Whole carbs provide things processed carbs never can:

1. **Fiber** slows sugar absorption, stabilizing blood sugar and feeding healthy gut bacteria.
2. **Nutrients** (B vitamins, magnesium, potassium) fuel enzymes, hormones, and repair systems.
3. **Phytochemicals** protect against cancer, inflammation, and aging.

An apple is not "just sugar." It's water, fiber, vitamin C, antioxidants, and healing compounds. Compare that to apple juice or candy — sugar stripped of its package.

The P53 Diet & Lifestyle: Carb Success

When I developed the **P53 Diet & Lifestyle**, one of its foundations was **emphasizing complex carbohydrates as the bulk of calories — 75 to 80%.**

People are often shocked by this. "Won't that make me fat? Won't that cause diabetes?" The opposite is true.

When calories come from beans, lentils, fruits, vegetables, potatoes, quinoa, and brown rice:

- **Weight normalizes.** The fiber and water content prevent overeating.
- **Blood sugar stabilizes.** Fiber slows glucose entry into the bloodstream.
- **Cholesterol drops.** Whole carbs are cholesterol-free and displace animal fats.

- **Energy rises.** Glucose becomes steady fuel instead of rollercoaster spikes.

Time and again, I've seen people thrive with this approach. They lose weight, reverse diabetes, lower blood pressure, and feel years younger. The "carb fear" vanishes once they experience real carbohydrates — the kind nature intended.

Breaking Down Sugar Addiction

Sugar doesn't just taste good — it acts like a drug.

When refined sugar hits the tongue, it rapidly floods the bloodstream, spiking glucose and lighting up the brain's reward system. Dopamine — the "feel-good" neurotransmitter — surges. The same brain circuits that respond to cocaine, nicotine, and alcohol light up when you eat cookies or drink soda.

That's why sugar is addictive. The more you eat, the more you crave.

- **Tolerance develops:** The brain reduces dopamine receptors, so you need more sugar for the same "hit."
- **Withdrawal appears:** Cut sugar suddenly and you may feel irritable, tired, or moody.
- **Cycle continues:** The rollercoaster of sugar highs and crashes leads to constant hunger and cravings.

This is not weakness. It is chemistry. Sugar hijacks the brain's natural pathways.

How to Break Free

The good news is that taste buds and brain chemistry can reset in just weeks:

- Replace soda with sparkling water and lemon.
- Swap candy for dates, figs, or bananas.

- Use whole fruits to sweeten oatmeal or smoothies.
- Add fiber (beans, vegetables, oats) to stabilize blood sugar and reduce cravings.

Over time, fruit begins to taste sweeter. Cravings shrink. Energy steadies. What once felt like an addiction loosens its grip.

The Low-Carb Lie

Low-carb diets have been fashionable for decades. Atkins, keto, paleo, carnivore — all promise quick weight loss. And yes, they sometimes deliver at first.

But here's why:

- Cutting carbs also cuts out junk food: sodas, pastries, white bread. Naturally, weight drops in the short term.
- Depleting glycogen (stored carbohydrate in muscles and liver) sheds water weight. This makes the scale look good — temporarily.

But the long-term effects tell a different story:

- **Nutrient loss:** Low-carb means cutting fruits, beans, and whole grains — the richest sources of fiber, antioxidants, and minerals.
- **High fat load:** To replace carbs, people eat meat, butter, cheese, and oils. This raises cholesterol and fuels heart disease and cancer.

- **Shorter lifespan:** Studies consistently show plant-rich, carb-rich diets correlate with longevity, while high animal fat and protein shorten it.

Low-carb is not sustainable. It may shrink your waistline briefly, but it weakens your terrain over time.

The Energy Connection

Carbohydrates are the body's **cleanest, most efficient fuel.**

- **Glucose** from whole carbs enters cells steadily, providing a smooth stream of energy.
- **Fat** is a backup fuel. It burns slowly and produces more metabolic waste.
- **Protein** is not designed for energy. Breaking it down for fuel strips muscles and stresses the liver and kidneys.

That's why endurance athletes "carb load." Muscles run on glycogen — stored carbohydrate. Without it, performance collapses. The brain too runs almost exclusively on glucose. Starve it, and you feel foggy, irritable, and slow.

When you eat fruit, beans, or sweet potatoes, you're giving your body the premium fuel it was designed for. That's why the **P53 Diet & Lifestyle thrives with 75–80% of calories from complex carbs.** The result is energy, clarity, and stamina.

Carbs, Cancer, and the Warburg Effect

One of the most powerful reasons to avoid refined sugar is its role in cancer. Cancer cells are metabolically abnormal. They prefer to ferment glucose into lactate — even when oxygen is available. This phenomenon is called the Warburg effect.

It means cancer cells are sugar addicts. The more simple glucose they get, the faster they grow.

But here's the distinction:

- **Refined sugars** (soda, candy, white flour) flood the bloodstream quickly, feeding tumors directly.
- **Complex carbs** (beans, fruit, whole grains) release glucose slowly, bundled with fiber, antioxidants, and phytochemicals that *fight cancer.*

For example:

- Beans provide resistant starch that nourishes gut bacteria, producing short-chain fatty acids that inhibit tumor growth.
- Fruits deliver vitamin C, carotenoids, and flavonoids — natural anti-cancer agents.
- Whole grains offer lignans and selenium, compounds that reduce oxidative stress and balance hormones.

So yes, cancer cells thrive on sugar — but the solution is not to cut all carbs. The solution is to cut refined sugar and load the body with **complex carbs that strengthen terrain and block cancer's pathways.**

Why Carbs Make Longevity Possible

Every long-lived culture on Earth bases their diet on carbohydrates — but not donuts and sodas. Their carbs are whole, complex, plant-based.

- Okinawans: sweet potatoes, rice, vegetables.
- Sardinians: beans, bread, greens.
- Nicoyans: corn tortillas, black beans, squash.
- Tarahumara: corn, beans, squash, wild greens.

These populations don't fear carbs. They embrace them. And their lifespans — with low rates of diabetes, heart disease, and cancer — prove the point.

The common thread: **complex carbs in abundance, refined sugar almost nonexistent.**

Stories That Make It Real
Robert's Low-Carb Crash

Robert tried a popular low-carb plan. At first, the weight dropped quickly — mostly water. But soon he was exhausted, constipated, and irritable. His cholesterol spiked, his blood sugar crept upward, and his doctor warned him about fatty liver. Frustrated, Robert gave the P53 approach a chance. He loaded up on beans, quinoa, sweet potatoes, fruit, and vegetables. Within weeks, his energy soared. Within months, his cholesterol fell and his liver healed. Carbs weren't his enemy — they were his medicine.

Elena's Banana Fear

Elena avoided bananas for years because of "too much sugar." Yet she battled constant cravings for cookies and chocolate. When she finally reintroduced bananas — along with berries, apples, and oranges — her cravings disappeared. The natural sugar in fruit gave her body what it needed, ending the cycle of junk food binges. Her digestion improved, her skin cleared, and she felt balanced again. The fruit she once feared became her healing food.

Derek the Runner

Derek loved long-distance running but often "hit the wall" mid-race. He thought eating more protein would fix it, but it didn't. Then he learned to carb-load with whole grains, beans, and starchy vegetables. His endurance doubled. He finished races strong, recovered faster, and realized what elite athletes already knew: **carbs are the body's premium fuel.**

Karen's Cancer Journey

Karen was diagnosed with breast cancer. Her oncologist told her to avoid sugar, but no one explained the difference between refined sugar and whole-food carbs. She cut fruit and whole grains, but still ate bread, cheese, and chicken. Her energy crashed, and she lost muscle. When she learned that complex carbs do not feed cancer the same way refined sugars do, she shifted to beans, greens, fruit, and brown rice. Her energy returned, her labs stabilized, and she felt strong enough to keep exercising during treatment.

These stories carry one message: **the source of the carbohydrate makes all the difference.**

Practical Carb Choices

Carbs don't need to be confusing. Here's a simple roadmap:

- **Best Carbs (Eat Daily):**
    - Fruits: apples, bananas, berries, oranges, grapes, mangoes.
    - Vegetables: sweet potatoes, squash, carrots, leafy greens.
    - Legumes: beans, lentils, chickpeas, peas.
    - Whole Grains: oats, brown rice, quinoa, barley, millet.
- **Middle Ground (Okay in Moderation):**

- Whole-grain breads, sprouted bread, whole-grain pasta, corn tortillas.
  - Lightly processed foods that still contain fiber and nutrients.
- **Avoid (Remove):**
  - Soda, candy, pastries, white bread, refined crackers, sugary cereals.
  - "Energy" drinks or bars loaded with added sugar.

Think of it this way: if it grew in nature and still looks close to how it grew, it's a healing carbohydrate. If it came from a factory in a shiny package, it's a harmful carbohydrate.

Expanded Key Takeaways

- **Not all carbs are equal.** Whole carbs heal. Refined carbs harm.
- **Refined sugar fuels disease.** Diabetes, obesity, cancer, and heart disease thrive on it.
- **Whole carbs build life.** Fiber stabilizes blood sugar, phytochemicals fight inflammation, nutrients fuel repair.
- **Longevity cultures thrive on carbs.** 60–80% of calories from plant-based carbs = lean bodies, long lives.
- **The P53 Diet & Lifestyle works.** Success comes from 75–80% of calories as complex carbs — beans, fruits, vegetables, and whole grains.
- **Carbs = clean energy.** They are the body's preferred fuel, while fats and protein are backups.

Action Steps

1. **Replace one sugary drink today.** Swap soda for water, sparkling water, or unsweetened tea.
2. **Add beans daily.** Lentils, black beans, or chickpeas add fiber, protein, and steady carbs.
3. **Eat fruit without fear.** Enjoy 2–4 servings daily to calm cravings and fuel energy.
4. **Choose whole grains.** Brown rice, oats, quinoa, or millet instead of white bread or pasta.
5. **Read labels.** Learn where sugar hides — in sauces, condiments, and "health" snacks.
6. **Make carbs 75–80% of your calories.** Let beans, whole grains, fruits, and vegetables form the base of your meals.

Closing Message

Carbs aren't the villain. Sugar isn't "evil" when it comes in fruit or sweet potatoes. The real enemy is refined, processed sugar masquerading as food.

The truth is simple: **your body runs on carbohydrates.** Every cell, every organ, every brain cell depends on glucose. The question is whether that glucose comes from candy bars or from beans and bananas.

In **Taste Versus Cancer**, I explained how sugar fuels tumors and inflammation.

This book keeps it simple: **don't fear carbs — fear refined sugar. Whole carbs are your body's best fuel.**

Choose beans over bacon. Brown rice over white bread. Fruit over candy. Your body will thank you with strength, clarity, and resilience.

Chapter 6

Proteins & Amino Acids: The Building Blocks

Protein is the superstar of modern nutrition. It's stamped on cereal boxes, splashed across yogurt labels, mixed into shakes and powders, and pushed in snack bars. Food marketers love protein because people fear deficiency. "Am I getting enough protein?" is one of the most common health questions — far more common than "Am I getting enough fiber, potassium, or magnesium?"

But here's the surprising truth: **protein deficiency is almost nonexistent in developed countries.** With so much food variety, nearly everyone easily meets their protein needs without trying.

The real danger isn't too little protein. It's too much — especially from animal sources.

Excess protein overstimulates growth pathways in the body, particularly a powerful hormone called **IGF-1 (Insulin-Like Growth Factor 1).** While IGF-1 is needed in childhood for growth and in adulthood for repair, too much acts like gasoline on a fire: fueling cancer, accelerating aging, and contributing to weight gain.

Whenever I order a plant-based meal, I get the same question: 'Do you want to add protein?' What most people don't realize is that every whole food — beans, grains, vegetables, nuts — already contains protein. The idea that you have to tack it on is a myth created by marketing, not biology.

What Protein Really Is

Protein is broken into amino acids, the building blocks of life. They form muscles, enzymes, hormones, neurotransmitters, and immune cells. Every organ and tissue in your body depends on amino acids.

There are 20 amino acids, and 9 are considered essential because the body cannot make them — they must come from food.

And here's the key: **every single essential amino acid is available in plants.**

The Incomplete Protein Myth

For decades, people believed plant proteins were "incomplete." This myth said that because some plants are lower in certain amino acids (like lysine or methionine), you had to eat animal foods to get the full set.

That was debunked years ago. Here's why:

- The body maintains an amino acid pool from all foods eaten across the day.
- Eat a variety of plants — beans, grains, nuts, seeds, and vegetables — and the body easily combines them into complete proteins.
- You don't need "protein combining" at the same meal. Your body is a **master chemist** that balances amino acids naturally.

As I explained in **Understanding Hormones, Enzymes, and Cell Receptors,** the human body is designed to assemble amino acids into the exact proteins needed, no matter the order or timing of intake.

You don't need meat for "complete" protein. You just need plants.

Animal Protein: Built with Baggage

Animal foods do deliver amino acids. But they also deliver a heavy burden:

- **Cholesterol** → clogs arteries.
- **Saturated fat** → fuels heart disease.
- **IGF-1 stimulation** → overstimulates growth pathways, fueling cancer and obesity.
- **Hormones and antibiotics** → disrupt balance and gut health.
- **Acid load** → leaches calcium from bones and stresses kidneys.

So while you get protein, you also get disease risk.

IGF-1: The Growth Hormone That Backfires

IGF-1 is a hormone your liver produces in response to protein intake — especially animal protein.

- In childhood, IGF-1 is essential for growth.
- In adulthood, small amounts help with repair.
- But chronically high IGF-1 keeps cells in a constant state of growth and division.

And that's dangerous. Why? Because uncontrolled cell growth is the definition of cancer.

High IGF-1 levels are linked to:

- **Breast cancer** (increased tumor growth and spread).
- **Prostate cancer** (faster progression).
- **Colorectal cancer** (higher risk).
- **Accelerated aging** (cells burn out faster).

And yes — weight gain. When IGF-1 is elevated, fat cells expand more easily, and insulin sensitivity decreases, leading to higher fat storage.

Animal protein is a direct stimulator of IGF-1. Plant protein is not. That's why high-meat diets often correlate with obesity and cancer, while plant-rich diets extend life.

Plant Protein: Clean and Complete

Plants provide every essential amino acid without the baggage.

- **Legumes**: beans, lentils, chickpeas.
- **Nuts and seeds**: hemp, chia, almonds, pumpkin seeds.
- **Grains**: quinoa, oats, brown rice, millet.
- **Vegetables**: broccoli, spinach, peas, even potatoes.

Together, these foods easily cover protein needs while also delivering fiber, antioxidants, vitamins, and minerals. Unlike animal protein, they do not overstimulate IGF-1, raise cholesterol, or create acid loads that weaken bones.

Plant protein builds strength without disease risk.

How Much Protein Do You Really Need?
The recommended daily intake is about **0.8 grams per kilogram of body weight.**

- For most people, that's 50–70 grams per day.
- This is easily met with whole plant foods.
- P53 Diet 1200 calorie plan is **38 grams per day.**

Example plant-based day:

- Oatmeal with chia = 10g
- Lentil soup = 18g
- Quinoa salad = 12g
- Almonds = 6g
- Beans and broccoli = 15g

Total = 61g — no animal foods, no powders. Just clean, balanced protein from plants.

IGF-1: When Growth Becomes Dangerous
One of the most overlooked problems with excess protein is its effect on **IGF-1 (Insulin-Like Growth Factor 1).**

Think of IGF-1 as the body's "grow" switch. In children, it's necessary — bones lengthen, muscles expand, cells divide rapidly. But in adults, constant stimulation of this pathway becomes harmful.

When IGF-1 is too high, it:

- **Drives cancer growth.** Cancer cells are like weeds; IGF-1 is the fertilizer that makes them spread faster.
- **Promotes weight gain.** High IGF-1 increases fat storage and reduces insulin sensitivity, encouraging belly fat.
- **Accelerates aging.** Cells divide faster, burn out sooner, and accumulate damage. People with lower IGF-1 levels consistently live longer.

Animal protein — especially from red meat, dairy, and eggs — spikes IGF-1. Plant protein does not. This is why people eating high-animal-protein diets often struggle with stubborn weight, while plant-based eaters maintain leaner bodies without trying.

Protein Powders: The Marketing Scam

Walk into any supplement store, and you'll find entire walls of protein powders. Whey, casein, collagen, soy isolate, pea protein — each promising strength, muscle, and "clean fuel."

But for most people, protein powders are unnecessary and sometimes harmful:

- **You already get enough protein.** Most people eating a variety of plant foods exceed the recommended 50–70 grams per day.
- **Powders are processed.** They strip away the natural package of fiber, antioxidants, and minerals.
- **Contaminants are common.** Studies find heavy metals (lead, arsenic, cadmium), pesticides, and microplastics in many powders.
- **They overstimulate IGF-1.** Whey and casein (from dairy) in particular spike IGF-1 levels dramatically.

Unless you're an elite athlete burning thousands of calories daily, powders are a marketing trick. Whole foods provide everything you need — cleaner, safer, and balanced.

The Strain of Excess Protein

Protein overload isn't just unnecessary — it damages the body.

- **Kidney Strain:** Excess protein increases nitrogen waste, forcing kidneys to work harder. Over time, this can worsen kidney disease or create it in vulnerable people.
- **Bone Loss:** Animal protein creates an acidic load. To buffer the acidity, the body pulls calcium from bones, weakening them over time. That's why high-dairy nations often have higher osteoporosis rates.
- **Dehydration:** High protein intake increases water loss through urine, stressing the body further.
- **Digestive Burden:** Heavy meat diets are linked to constipation and gut imbalance, since they lack fiber.

Ironically, the very foods people eat for "strength" slowly weaken the organs that support them.

Plant Protein and Longevity

The longest-lived people on earth — from Okinawa to Sardinia — don't chase protein shakes or eat steak every day. They eat **moderate protein from plants.**

- **Okinawans:** Get protein mainly from soy (tofu, miso), sweet potatoes, vegetables, and legumes.
- **Sardinians:** Rely on beans, bread, and greens for protein.

- **Adventists (California):** One of the healthiest populations in the U.S., thriving on beans, nuts, and grains.

In each case, protein makes up a normal, moderate percentage of calories — mostly plant-based. The result: long lives, low rates of cancer, and lean, strong bodies well into old age.

By contrast, high-animal-protein diets shorten lifespan. Studies consistently show:

- People eating the most animal protein have the **highest cancer and heart disease risk.**
- People eating the most plant protein have the **lowest risk of early death.**

It's not protein itself that's the problem. It's the source.

Stories That Make It Real
Jason's Gym Obsession

Jason was a 35-year-old weightlifter who lived on chicken, steak, and whey protein shakes. His goal was muscle mass, but his cholesterol soared, he developed acid reflux, and despite hours at the gym, his waistline expanded. When he switched to plant-based proteins — lentils, quinoa, tempeh, and beans — his body transformed. He lost fat, gained lean muscle, and his acid reflux vanished. His doctor was astonished when his cholesterol normalized without medication. Jason learned that building strength didn't require animal protein or powders. It required clean fuel.

Martha's Fear of Weakness

Martha, in her 50s, feared going plant-based because she thought she'd "waste away without meat." Instead, her joints ached, her digestion was sluggish, and her doctor warned her about early osteoporosis. When she shifted to beans, almonds, chia seeds, and leafy greens, she was shocked by how strong and light she felt. Within months, her bone scans stabilized, her digestion improved, and she had more stamina on hikes than she did in her 40s. Far from wasting away, she thrived.

Andre's Protein Powder Addiction

Andre worked long hours and relied on protein shakes for "quick nutrition." But constant bloating, kidney discomfort, and fatigue plagued him. A friend urged him to ditch the powders for whole foods. He swapped shakes for chickpeas, oats, nuts, and vegetables. His digestion healed, his energy soared, and bloodwork showed his kidneys were no longer under strain. Andre realized protein powders were part of the problem, not the solution.

Sofia's Cancer Scare

Sofia's father had died from prostate cancer, and when she learned about IGF-1, she realized her heavy meat-and-dairy diet was putting her at risk. She gradually replaced meat with lentils and dairy with soy yogurt and almond milk. Over time, she lost weight, her blood sugar stabilized, and her IGF-1 levels dropped into a safer range. She felt empowered knowing her food choices weren't fueling the same disease that claimed her father.

These stories echo the same lesson: **protein is essential, but the *source* of protein shapes your health destiny.**

Practical Protein Choices

If you want strength without the baggage, here's how to do it:

- **Base Every Meal on Plants:** Make beans, lentils, quinoa, or tofu the centerpiece.
- **Snack Smart:** Almonds, walnuts, pumpkin seeds, or hummus with vegetables.
- **Mix and Match:** Rice and beans, pita with hummus, lentils with sweet potatoes — simple meals that naturally cover amino acid needs.
- **Use Vegetables as Protein Boosters:** Broccoli, spinach, peas, and potatoes all add protein while also providing fiber and micronutrients.
- **Ditch the Powder:** Unless you're training like an Olympic athlete, whole foods are enough.

You'll quickly discover that hitting 50–70 grams a day is effortless with plants.

Expanded Key Takeaways

- **Protein deficiency is rare.** In developed nations, people easily meet needs.
- **Excess animal protein is dangerous.** It overstimulates IGF-1, fueling cancer, weight gain, and accelerated aging.
- **Plant protein is complete.** All nine essential amino acids are available in plants.
- **Protein powders are unnecessary.** They often contain contaminants and overstimulate IGF-1.
- **Excess protein strains kidneys and bones.** Acid load weakens skeletons, while nitrogen waste stresses kidneys.
- **Plant protein supports longevity.** Blue Zones prove that moderate, plant-based protein correlates with long life and low disease.

Action Steps

1. **Add Beans Daily.** Black beans, lentils, chickpeas — your best protein allies.
2. **Swap Meat for Quinoa or Tofu.** Both are versatile, protein-rich, and nutrient-packed.
3. **Snack on Seeds.** A handful of pumpkin or chia adds amino acids plus minerals.
4. **Skip the Powders.** Replace a shake with a bean soup or lentil salad.
5. **Track One Day.** Count your protein intake from plants — you'll be surprised at how easily it adds up.

Closing Message

Protein is not the problem. The obsession with it is.

You don't need meat, eggs, or powders to get enough protein. You need plants. Every essential amino acid is found in them — without the baggage of cholesterol, saturated fat, hormones, antibiotics, or acid loads.

The real danger of animal protein is its effect on **IGF-1.** When overstimulated, IGF-1 accelerates cancer, drives weight gain, and shortens lifespan. Plant protein, by contrast, provides what you need without overstimulating growth. It builds strength without fueling disease.

Chapter 7

Fruit: Nature's Sweetest Medicine

Before there were grocery stores, refrigerators, or restaurants, there was fruit.

On every continent, early humans survived and thrived on fruit. It was the original fast food: colorful, portable, ready to eat, and loaded with water, fiber, and nutrients. Peel it, bite it, enjoy it.

And yet today, fruit is under attack.

- Fad diets warn about "too much sugar in fruit."
- Social media influencers tell people to avoid bananas, mangoes, or grapes.
- People fear fruit while eating protein bars full of chemicals.

It's madness.

Here's the truth: **fruit is one of the most powerful healing foods on Earth.**

Why Fruit Heals

Fruit isn't just sweet. It's a complete package of health.

- **Vitamins:** Vitamin C (immune protection, collagen formation), folate (DNA repair, pregnancy health), beta-carotene (vision, antioxidant protection).
- **Minerals:** Potassium (blood pressure balance), magnesium (muscle and nerve function), calcium (bone strength).
- **Fiber:** Slows sugar absorption, improves digestion, lowers cholesterol, stabilizes weight.
- **Antioxidants:** Polyphenols, anthocyanins, carotenoids, flavonoids — compounds that fight free radicals and repair cellular damage.
- **Water:** Built-in hydration in perfect balance with electrolytes.

Every bite of fruit is like swallowing a pharmacy of healing molecules — designed not in a lab, but by nature.

Fruit doesn't just prevent disease. It actively rebuilds and protects the body.

The Sugar Myth

One of the most persistent lies about fruit is that its sugar is the same as candy or soda.

That's false.

- **Refined sugar** = empty calories that spike blood sugar, overwhelm insulin, and fuel disease.
- **Fruit sugar** = naturally packaged with fiber, water, antioxidants, and phytochemicals that protect against those very effects.

An apple doesn't hit your system like candy. The fiber slows digestion. The antioxidants protect cells. The phytochemicals boost immunity.

No one gets sick from eating too many oranges. But plenty of people get sick from soda.

Fruit and Longevity

Every long-lived culture on Earth eats fruit daily.

- **Okinawa (Japan):** Purple sweet potatoes, citrus, and seasonal fruits.
- **Ikaria (Greece):** Figs, grapes, pomegranates.
- **Nicoya (Costa Rica):** Bananas, papayas, oranges.
- **Hunza (Pakistan):** Apricots, mulberries, apples.

Fruit isn't a garnish or a snack. It's a staple. These cultures didn't fear fruit. They celebrated it. And the results? They had some of the lowest rates of chronic disease and some of the longest lifespans in the world.

The Cancer Connection

Fruit isn't just about vitamins and sweetness. It's one of the most powerful cancer-preventive foods.

- **Berries** (blueberries, raspberries, strawberries, blackberries): Loaded with anthocyanins that protect DNA and block tumor growth.
- **Grapes and pomegranates:** Contain resveratrol and ellagic acid, both known to slow cancer spread and trigger cancer cell self-destruction.
- **Citrus fruits:** Rich in limonene, which detoxifies carcinogens and supports liver function.
- **Apples and pears:** Provide quercetin and flavonoids that lower inflammation and reduce oxidative stress.

In **Taste Versus Cancer,** I documented study after study showing fruit reduces cancer risk. Researchers consistently find that people who eat more fruit have lower rates of nearly every major cancer.

Fruit isn't just safe — it's protective.

Fruit for Energy

Fruit is the cleanest, most efficient energy source you can eat.

It digests easily, hydrates as it nourishes, and delivers glucose steadily to muscles and the brain. That's why athletes are rediscovering fruit as performance fuel.

- **Bananas, dates, and oranges** outperform artificial gels and processed "energy" snacks.
- Natural sugar, balanced with fiber and potassium, provides sustainable energy instead of spikes and crashes.

For the everyday person, fruit gives clarity of mind and steady fuel throughout the day. It's no coincidence that when people eat fruit in the morning, they feel light and energized instead of sluggish.

Weight and Fruit

One of the greatest myths is that fruit causes weight gain. The truth? Fruit eaters consistently weigh less.

- Fiber fills the stomach, creating satiety.
- Nutrients satisfy cellular needs, reducing cravings.
- Water dilutes calories — an apple or orange provides only 60–100 calories while filling the stomach more than a candy bar.

Studies repeatedly show higher fruit consumption is linked to lower body weight, lower waist circumference, and reduced obesity rates.

Fruit doesn't make you fat. It makes you full.

Fruit's Healing Compounds in Depth

Fruit is more than a source of vitamins and fiber. Each variety carries its own pharmacy of phytochemicals — natural plant compounds with profound effects on human health.

- **Polyphenols:** Found in grapes, apples, pears, and berries. These compounds reduce oxidative stress and inflammation, lowering risk of heart disease and cancer.
- **Anthocyanins:** Give berries, cherries, and purple grapes their deep colors. They repair DNA damage, improve blood vessel function, and block tumor growth.
- **Carotenoids:** Found in oranges, mangoes, apricots, and papayas. These protect eyesight, boost immunity, and help regulate gene expression in ways that fight cancer.
- **Flavonoids:** Present in citrus fruits, apples, and plums. They calm inflammation and strengthen immune defenses.
- **Ellagic acid & Resveratrol:** From pomegranates and grapes. They slow the spread of cancer and even help trigger apoptosis (programmed cancer cell death).

Every piece of fruit is like a personalized prescription from nature. One apple, one handful of berries, one slice of watermelon — each delivers compounds that modern science is still trying to replicate in pills.

But here's the key: **fruit isn't just one nutrient.** It's a *synergy*. The fiber, water, vitamins, and phytochemicals work together in ways that isolated extracts never can.

Fruit and Gut Health

Your gut is home to trillions of bacteria — your microbiome — which shapes digestion, immunity, mood, and even disease risk. Fruit is one of the best foods you can feed it.

- **Prebiotic fiber** in apples, bananas, pears, and berries feeds good bacteria.
- **Polyphenols** in grapes, blueberries, and pomegranates nourish beneficial microbes while suppressing harmful ones.
- **Short-chain fatty acids (SCFAs):** Produced when gut bacteria ferment fruit fiber. SCFAs lower inflammation, strengthen the gut lining, and protect against colon cancer.

People who eat more fruit have greater microbiome diversity — a hallmark of better health. In contrast, diets heavy in animal foods reduce microbial diversity, fostering inflammation and disease.

Fruit doesn't just nourish you — it nourishes your *internal ecosystem*.

Fruit and Immunity

Fruit also strengthens the immune system in multiple ways:

- **Vitamin C** (citrus, kiwi, strawberries) enhances white blood cell activity.

- **Carotenoids** (mango, papaya, apricots) modulate immune signaling.
- **Flavonoids** (oranges, apples, grapes) reduce inflammation that weakens immunity.
- **Fiber** regulates blood sugar, preventing immune suppression from sugar spikes.

When people replace processed snacks with fruit, they often notice fewer colds, faster healing, and greater resilience. It isn't magic — it's the body finally getting the compounds it needs.

Juice vs. Whole Fruit

Many people think drinking fruit juice is the same as eating fruit. It isn't.

- **Whole fruit:** Fiber slows digestion, preventing sugar spikes. Water dilutes calories. Nutrients are intact.
- **Juice:** The fiber is stripped away. Sugar is concentrated. A glass of orange juice = 4 oranges, but without the natural balance.

The result: juice floods the bloodstream with sugar in ways whole fruit never does.

That doesn't mean juice has zero value — fresh-squeezed juice still provides vitamins and phytochemicals. But it should be an occasional treat, not a daily staple. Whole fruit always wins.

The Psychology of Fruit Fear

Why do so many people fear fruit?

It's the result of decades of diet culture and misinformation:

- **Low-carb diets** lump fruit together with soda and candy, ignoring fiber and nutrients.
- **Fitness influencers** warn against bananas or grapes while selling protein shakes.
- **Food industry marketing** promotes "protein bars" and "low-carb snacks" over nature's simplest food.

The irony? Nobody gets diabetes from eating blueberries. Nobody becomes obese from oranges. Yet millions suffer from sodas, pastries, and candy.

Fruit fear is a myth that benefits industries selling packaged products. The science says the opposite: **fruit is protective.**

Fruit as Everyday Medicine

Imagine if doctors prescribed fruit the way they prescribe pills:

- **Blueberries** for memory and brain health.
- **Oranges** for immune support.
- **Apples** for cholesterol reduction.
- **Bananas** for digestion and heart health.
- **Pomegranates** for cancer prevention.

If fruit came in a pill, it would be the best-selling drug of all time. Instead, it grows on trees — and too many people ignore it.

Stories That Make It Real
Daniel's Sweet Tooth Fix

Daniel had battled sugar cravings for years. Candy bars and sodas were his daily comfort. He thought fruit was "too sugary," so he avoided it. When his doctor warned him about prediabetes, he finally tried a different approach: replacing candy with grapes, apples, and pears. To his surprise, his cravings vanished. He didn't miss candy anymore because fruit satisfied him naturally. Within months, his blood sugar stabilized, his weight dropped, and his energy returned. His sweet tooth wasn't the problem. The *wrong* sugar was.

Marisol's Digestion Dilemma

Marisol avoided fruit for years because she thought it upset her stomach. But her real issue was processed food. When she reintroduced bananas, papaya, and kiwi, her digestion healed. The soluble fiber soothed her gut, the enzymes in papaya aided breakdown of proteins, and the natural hydration eased constipation. Her stomach pains disappeared — fruit wasn't her problem. It was her solution.

Paul the Runner

Paul trained for marathons and relied on energy gels and sports drinks. Yet he often hit the wall midway through races. A coach suggested bananas, dates, and oranges instead. The difference was night and day. Fruit fueled his muscles better, kept him hydrated, and prevented the sugar crashes he had with processed gels. His times improved, his recovery sped up, and he realized athletes don't need chemical carbs. They need fruit.

Anita's Cancer Prevention Shift

Anita had a family history of breast cancer. She learned that berries, grapes, and citrus were loaded with phytochemicals that protect DNA and block tumor growth. She made fruit central to every meal — berries on oatmeal, citrus in salads, grapes as snacks. Over the years, her weight stabilized, her cholesterol dropped, and her doctors marveled at her resilience. For Anita, fruit wasn't just food. It was daily prevention.

These stories reveal a truth often buried by diet fads: **fruit heals in ways no supplement, powder, or processed food ever could.**

Practical Ways to Eat More Fruit

Adding more fruit doesn't have to be complicated. Try these strategies:

1. **Start Your Day with Fruit.** A smoothie, oatmeal with berries, or simply an apple gives clean energy to begin the day.
2. **Snack Smart.** Carry bananas, apples, or oranges instead of chips or bars. Portable, filling, and nourishing.
3. **Add Fruit to Meals.** Toss berries into salads, top grains with pomegranate seeds, or use mango salsa on beans and rice.
4. **Dessert Upgrade.** Replace cakes or cookies with grapes, melon, or baked apples with cinnamon.
5. **Seasonal Rotation.** Choose fruit that's in season for maximum nutrients and flavor. Strawberries in summer, citrus in winter, apples in fall.

With small shifts, fruit can reclaim its place as a cornerstone of daily life.

Juice vs. Whole Fruit (Revisited)

It's worth repeating: **whole fruit wins every time.**

- Juice delivers sugar without fiber, making it easy to overconsume.
- Whole fruit delivers balance — fiber, water, antioxidants, and satiety.

An orange is medicine. A glass of orange juice is concentrated sugar. Choose nature's version.

Expanded Key Takeaways

- **Fruit is medicine.** It's not sugar to fear, but a healing food to embrace.
- **Nutrient powerhouse.** Vitamins, minerals, fiber, and phytochemicals protect DNA, repair cells, and prevent disease.
- **Fruit does not cause weight gain.** Studies show fruit eaters are leaner and healthier.
- **The sugar myth is false.** Fruit sugar is balanced by fiber and nutrients, unlike refined sugar.
- **Longevity cultures prove the point.** Every long-lived community eats fruit daily.
- **Juice ≠ fruit.** Whole fruit is the real medicine.

Action Steps

1. **Replace one processed snack with fruit today.**
2. **Start breakfast with fruit.** Add berries, bananas, or citrus.
3. **Eat at least 3–5 servings of fruit daily.** Spread it across meals and snacks.
4. **Experiment with variety.** Try exotic fruits like dragonfruit, papaya, or passionfruit to expand your nutrient spectrum.
5. **End dinner with fruit instead of dessert.** Satisfy the sweet tooth naturally.

Closing Message

Fruit isn't dangerous. It isn't "too much sugar." Those are lies created by diet fads and processed food industries.

The truth is simple: **fruit is nature's sweetest medicine.** The more you eat, the better you live.

In ***The P53 Diet & Lifestyle,*** I emphasized fruit as central to prevention — not just for energy, but for disease reversal. In ***Taste Versus Cancer,*** I documented how fruit's phytochemicals — anthocyanins, carotenoids, resveratrol, limonene — block tumors, repair DNA, and protect cells.

This book keeps it simple: **fruit heals.**

Choose berries over candy, grapes over soda, oranges over supplements. Every piece of fruit is a gift of life from nature, waiting to strengthen you.

The truth is clear: **the path to energy, immunity, and longevity is sweet — and it grows on trees.**

Chapter 8

Vegetables: The Unsung Heroes of Health

Ask most people their favorite food, and you'll hear pizza, burgers, or pasta. Rarely will you hear broccoli, kale, or spinach. Vegetables don't get the glory, but they are the backbone of health. Quietly, they do the heavy lifting — supplying nutrients, repairing damage, and protecting life.

Every culture with long-lived people eats vegetables daily. Whether from gardens, wild fields, or local markets, vegetables form the nutritional base of humanity's healthiest diets.

While meat, dairy, or sugar get more attention, vegetables are the steady protectors that prevent disease and extend life.

Why Vegetables Heal
Vegetables deliver a pharmacy of nutrients in every bite:

- **Vitamins:** A (eye and immune health), C (collagen and immunity), K (blood clotting and bone strength), folate (DNA repair and pregnancy health).

- **Minerals:** Magnesium (muscle relaxation, enzyme function), potassium (blood pressure balance), calcium (bones and nerves), iron (oxygen transport).
- **Fiber:** Cleans the digestive tract, lowers cholesterol, regulates blood sugar, and feeds gut bacteria.
- **Antioxidants:** Thousands of compounds — flavonoids, carotenoids, glucosinolates — that reduce inflammation, neutralize free radicals, and repair damage.

Unlike pills, vegetables provide synergy — dozens of compounds working together. That's why vegetable nutrients are more effective than supplements. They arrive packaged with cofactors, enzymes, and fiber designed for human biology.

The Cancer Connection
Vegetables are cancer's worst enemy.

- **Cruciferous vegetables (broccoli, kale, cauliflower, Brussels sprouts):** Contain sulforaphane, a compound that activates detox enzymes, protects DNA, and blocks tumor growth.
- **Carrots and sweet potatoes:** Rich in carotenoids like beta-carotene, which protect the lungs and skin from oxidative damage.
- **Onions, garlic, leeks:** Packed with sulfur compounds that detoxify carcinogens and reduce inflammation.
- **Spinach, kale, collards:** Loaded with lutein and zeaxanthin for eye health, plus folate for DNA repair.

In **Taste Versus Cancer,** I showed how each family of vegetables carries unique shields against disease. No single pill or drug can replicate the broad cancer protection that vegetables provide naturally.

The Color Code

One of the simplest ways to understand vegetables is to look at their colors. Each color signals different healing compounds:

- **Green:** Chlorophyll detoxifies, magnesium calms muscles, calcium strengthens bones. Examples: kale, spinach, broccoli.
- **Orange/Yellow:** Beta-carotene boosts immunity and protects vision. Examples: carrots, squash, sweet potatoes.
- **Red:** Lycopene protects the heart and prostate. Examples: tomatoes, red peppers.
- **Purple/Blue:** Anthocyanins shield the brain, improving memory and lowering dementia risk. Examples: eggplant, purple cabbage, blueberries.
- **White:** Sulfur compounds reduce inflammation and enhance immunity. Examples: onions, garlic, cauliflower.

A colorful plate isn't just pretty — it's a medicine chest.

Vegetables for Weight and Energy

Vegetables are naturally low in calories and high in nutrients. That means you can eat a large volume without gaining weight. They fill you up with fiber and water, not fat and sugar.

This is why plant-based diets succeed. They satisfy hunger while reducing calorie load. People who switch to vegetable-rich diets almost always lose weight — not because they eat less, but because they eat better.

Vegetables also provide steady energy. Unlike processed foods that spike and crash blood sugar, vegetables release glucose slowly, stabilizing energy throughout the day.

Vegetables and the Gut

Your gut bacteria thrive on vegetable fiber. Without it, the microbiome weakens, inflammation rises, and immunity collapses. With it, balance and resilience return.

- **Prebiotic fiber** in onions, garlic, asparagus, and leeks feeds beneficial bacteria.
- **Fermentable fiber** in beans, peas, and carrots produces short-chain fatty acids (SCFAs) that reduce colon cancer risk.
- **Polyphenols** in leafy greens and crucifers shape a healthier microbial balance.

The gut is the frontline of health, and vegetables are its best defense.

Cooking vs. Raw

One of the common debates is whether vegetables are healthier raw or cooked. The answer? Both matter. Each method unlocks different benefits.

- **Raw Vegetables**
  - Preserve enzymes that aid digestion.
  - Retain delicate nutrients like vitamin C and some B vitamins.
  - Offer maximum hydration and crisp fiber for gut health.
  - Best sources: leafy greens, cucumbers, peppers, carrots, lettuce, sprouts.

- **Cooked Vegetables**
  - Break down cell walls, releasing compounds otherwise locked inside.
  - Increase availability of antioxidants like lycopene (tomatoes) and beta-carotene (carrots, sweet potatoes).
  - Make cruciferous vegetables easier to digest while still delivering sulforaphane.
  - Heat neutralizes certain anti-nutrients (like oxalates in spinach), boosting calcium and iron absorption.

The key isn't choosing one over the other — it's **variety.** Eat some vegetables raw for freshness, crunch, and delicate vitamins. Eat some cooked to unlock deeper, fat-soluble compounds. A diet rich in both ensures maximum benefit.

More Disease-Fighting Compounds

Vegetables contain a vast library of phytochemicals, many only discovered in the past few decades. Science is still catching up to what cultures have known for centuries: vegetables prevent disease.

- **Sulforaphane (broccoli, kale, Brussels sprouts):** Stimulates detox enzymes that neutralize carcinogens, slows tumor growth, and protects against DNA mutations.
- **Lycopene (tomatoes, red peppers):** Reduces prostate cancer risk and supports cardiovascular health.

- **Beta-carotene (carrots, pumpkins, sweet potatoes):** Protects the lungs, eyes, and skin.
- **Lutein & Zeaxanthin (leafy greens, corn):** Defend against macular degeneration and vision loss.
- **Allicin (garlic, onions):** Potent anti-inflammatory and antimicrobial compound that lowers blood pressure and cholesterol and has been shown to induce apoptosis on 7 different cancer cell lines.
- **Indoles & Isothiocyanates (crucifers):** Balance hormones, reduce breast cancer risk, and help eliminate excess estrogen.

Each vegetable family brings its own arsenal. Together, they cover nearly every major disease pathway — cancer, heart disease, diabetes, neurodegeneration.

Vegetables in Longevity Cultures

The world's longest-lived people — often called the Blue Zones — treat vegetables as daily essentials, not optional sides.

- **Okinawa, Japan:** Bitter melon, sweet potatoes, and leafy greens form the foundation of meals. Their diet is ~70% complex carbohydrates with vegetables at the center.
- **Ikaria, Greece:** Wild greens like dandelion and fennel are staples, eaten daily in soups and stews.
- **Sardinia, Italy:** Families maintain gardens filled with tomatoes, beans, cabbage, onions, and kale.
- **Nicoya, Costa Rica:** Meals combine beans, corn, squash, and tropical vegetables like chayote.
- **Loma Linda, California (Adventists):** Plant-based diets rich in vegetables drive some of the longest lifespans in the U.S.

Across every region, vegetables are central. They aren't supplements, add-ons, or "diet foods." They are cultural anchors of nourishment and longevity.

Why Western Diets Undervalue Vegetables

Despite overwhelming evidence, many Western diets minimize vegetables. Why?

- **Marketing:** Meat, dairy, and processed foods dominate advertising. Vegetables don't have billion-dollar marketing campaigns.
- **Convenience:** Processed foods are faster, packaged, and engineered for taste. Vegetables require washing, chopping, and preparation.
- **Cultural Habits:** Meals are designed around meat as the centerpiece, with vegetables as sides or garnishes.
- **Misinformation:** Fad diets demonize starchy vegetables (like potatoes or corn), painting them as "bad carbs."

The result: Most Americans eat far below the recommended intake of vegetables. This deficiency quietly fuels obesity, cancer, heart disease, and diabetes.

By reframing vegetables as the foundation, not the garnish, we reclaim the power they've always offered.

Stories That Make It Real
Carlos's Blood Pressure Breakthrough

Carlos, a 52-year-old accountant, struggled with high blood pressure for years. His doctor prescribed medication, but his numbers barely budged. He admitted he barely ate vegetables — maybe a slice of tomato on a burger. At his wife's urging, he began adding salads with leafy greens, cucumbers, and peppers to every meal. Within months, his blood pressure dropped so much that his doctor reduced his medication. Carlos realized it wasn't a pill his body was missing — it was plants.

Janelle's Cholesterol Change

Janelle believed dairy and chicken were "healthy proteins." Vegetables were an afterthought. When her cholesterol numbers spiked, she faced the prospect of statins. Instead, she filled her meals with kale, broccoli, Brussels sprouts, and beans. Six months later, her cholesterol dropped over 40 points — without medication. Her doctor was stunned. Janelle wasn't just lowering cholesterol; she was nourishing her entire system.

Marcus's Energy Shift

Marcus lived on fast food and processed carbs. He was overweight, sluggish, and often sick. When he swapped fries and burgers for roasted vegetables, stir-fries, and soups loaded with carrots, kale, onions, and garlic, his transformation was dramatic. He lost weight, regained his energy, and even noticed clearer skin. Vegetables didn't just change his health markers — they changed his life.

Helen's Cancer Recovery Support

Helen underwent treatment for colon cancer. Alongside medical care, she committed to eating cruciferous vegetables daily: broccoli, cauliflower, and kale. The sulforaphane and antioxidants supported her immune system, helped her tolerate treatment better, and kept her blood counts strong. Her doctors encouraged her plant-rich diet, noting her resilience. Helen credits vegetables with helping her not just survive, but recover with strength.

These stories share one lesson: **vegetables are medicine in disguise.**

Practical Ways to Eat More Vegetables

Adding vegetables doesn't have to feel like punishment. With creativity, they can become the most enjoyable part of meals.

1. **Start Your Day with Greens.** Add spinach or kale to smoothies. Toss vegetables into tofu scrambles or breakfast bowls.
2. **Double the Side.** Instead of a small scoop, make vegetables half your plate at lunch and dinner.
3. **Keep Them Visible.** Wash and chop carrots, peppers, or cucumbers so they're ready for snacking.
4. **Upgrade Your Favorites.** Add mushrooms and spinach to pasta, bell peppers and zucchini to tacos, cauliflower to curry.
5. **Roast for Flavor.** Roasting brings out natural sweetness in carrots, Brussels sprouts, and beets.
6. **Flavor Naturally.** Use lemon juice, garlic, herbs, and spices instead of oil or heavy sauces.
7. **Try New Varieties.** Experiment with bok choy, fennel, or rainbow chard to keep meals exciting.

The key is making vegetables the centerpiece, not the side dish.

Expanded Key Takeaways

- **Vegetables are the backbone of health.** They deliver vitamins, minerals, fiber, and thousands of antioxidants.

- **They are cancer's worst enemy.** Crucifers, carotenoids, and sulfur compounds protect DNA and block tumor growth.
- **Colors matter.** Each color family signals unique protective compounds. A rainbow plate = maximum protection.
- **Vegetables support gut health.** Fiber and polyphenols feed good bacteria and strengthen immunity.
- **Both raw and cooked are essential.** Each preparation unlocks different nutrients.
- **Vegetables support weight balance.** High nutrients + low calories = natural satiety and energy.
- **Longevity cultures thrive on vegetables.** From Okinawa to Sardinia, vegetables are staples, not garnishes.

Action Steps

1. **Fill half your plate with vegetables at dinner.** Make them the foundation, not the afterthought.
2. **Try one new vegetable this week.** Variety ensures a wider spectrum of nutrients.
3. **Eat leafy greens daily.** Kale, spinach, collards, or arugula — rotate them for diversity.
4. **Replace one processed snack with cut vegetables.** Carrots, cucumbers, peppers, or celery with hummus.
5. **Cook creatively.** Soups, stir-fries, curries, and salads all showcase vegetables in delicious ways.

Closing Message

Vegetables don't get the spotlight, but they are the quiet heroes of health. They repair damage, strengthen defenses, and protect life at its core.

The truth is simple: **the more vegetables you eat, the longer and better you'll live.**

In *The P53 Diet & Lifestyle,* I emphasized vegetables as foundations of a healing diet. In *Taste Versus Cancer*, I detailed how crucifers, carotenoids, and sulfur compounds block disease at the cellular level.

This book simplifies the message: **vegetables aren't garnish — they're essential.**

Fill your plate with color. Celebrate the rainbow. Every bite of broccoli, carrot, or kale is not just food — it's prevention, energy, and life.

Chapter 9

Legumes: The Longevity Food

They don't look glamorous. They don't have celebrity endorsements or shiny packaging. But beans, lentils, peas, and chickpeas may be the single most powerful food for long life.

Every long-lived culture on Earth eats legumes daily. From Okinawa to Sardinia to Costa Rica, beans are the backbone of meals. If there's one food you should eat every day for health, it's legumes.

Why Legumes Heal

Legumes pack more nutrition per calorie than almost any other food group.

- **Protein:** 15–20 grams per cup, with all essential amino acids when combined with grains like rice or corn.
- **Fiber:** Both soluble and insoluble, feeding the gut, slowing sugar absorption, lowering cholesterol, and sweeping out toxins.

- **Minerals:** Iron (oxygen transport), magnesium (nerve and muscle function), potassium (blood pressure regulation), zinc (immune health).
- **Vitamins:** Folate (DNA repair and fetal development), B vitamins (metabolism and energy).
- **Phytochemicals:** Isoflavones, saponins, and antioxidants that fight inflammation, balance hormones, and block cancer pathways.

Few foods deliver as much nutrition for so few calories. A single cup of lentils or black beans gives the body protein, minerals, fiber, and healing compounds in one affordable package.

The Longevity Connection

In every Blue Zone — regions where people live the longest, healthiest lives — beans are eaten daily.

- **Okinawa, Japan:** Soybeans in tofu, miso, natto, and edamame are staples.
- **Nicoya, Costa Rica:** Black beans with corn tortillas form the foundation of meals.
- **Sardinia, Italy:** Fava beans, chickpeas, and lentil soups fuel shepherds and families.
- **Ikaria, Greece:** Lentils, chickpeas, and wild greens appear in daily stews and salads.
- **Loma Linda, California (Adventists):** Beans are central in vegetarian diets that lead to some of the longest lifespans in the U.S.

In each culture, beans are not a side dish. They're a staple food. And the people who eat them live longer, stronger, and freer of disease.

The Protein Myth Busted

Many people worry about protein on plant-based diets. But legumes end that worry.

- One cup of lentils has as much protein as three eggs — but without cholesterol, hormones, or saturated fat.
- Pair beans with rice or corn, and you cover all essential amino acids — a complete protein.
- Beans are also rich in lysine, an amino acid sometimes limited in grains. Together, beans and grains are the perfect match.

Animal protein comes with baggage. Bean protein comes **clean.**

The Cancer Connection

In **Taste Versus Cancer,** I highlighted how legumes protect against cancer. The science is clear:

- **Isoflavones in soy** block estrogen-driven cancers, reducing risk of breast and prostate cancer.
- **Fiber in beans** binds toxins and waste products in the gut, lowering colon cancer risk.
- **Antioxidants** in lentils, chickpeas, and kidney beans neutralize free radicals before they damage DNA.
- **Saponins and phytates** inhibit tumor growth by slowing cell division in malignant cells.

Populations that eat beans consistently have lower cancer rates. Legumes don't just feed the body — they protect it at the cellular level.

Weight and Satiety

Beans are among the **most filling foods on Earth.**

- Fiber slows digestion and stabilizes blood sugar.
- Protein provides steady fuel and reduces cravings.
- Nutrients satisfy the body's true needs, preventing overeating.

That's why people who eat more beans weigh less. Instead of spiking appetite, beans calm it. Instead of driving weight gain, beans encourage balance.

The Gut-Healing Power

Your gut bacteria thrive on bean fiber. When they ferment it, they produce **short-chain fatty acids** (SCFAs) — powerful compounds that:

- Reduce colon and systemic inflammation.
- Strengthen the gut lining, preventing leaky gut.
- Improve immunity by training immune cells in the gut.
- Even influence brain health, lowering depression and anxiety.

Yes, beans support mental health through the gut-brain connection.

Gas at first? That's often just the microbiome adjusting. Start slow, rinse canned beans, cook thoroughly, and within weeks, your digestion strengthens.

Busting the Myths About Beans

Despite their track record, beans and legumes face plenty of myths. Let's set the record straight.

1. "Beans cause gas."

It's true that some people experience bloating or gas when they first increase bean intake. This happens because beans are rich in fermentable fibers — the kind your gut bacteria *love*. As bacteria adjust and multiply, they ferment the fiber into beneficial short-chain fatty acids (SCFAs). With time, the gas decreases and digestion strengthens.

Tips to minimize discomfort:

- Start small — ¼ to ½ cup per day — and increase gradually.
- Rinse canned beans to remove some of the oligosaccharides that cause gas.
- Cook beans thoroughly with spices like cumin, fennel, or ginger to aid digestion.

Gas isn't a "problem." It's a sign your gut bacteria are getting stronger.

2. "Soy is dangerous."

Few foods are as misunderstood as soy. The fear largely comes from confusion about phytoestrogens, the plant compounds found in soy. Some worry they act like estrogen and stimulate cancer. The truth is more nuanced — and more protective.

- Soy isoflavones don't act exactly like human estrogen. They preferentially bind to estrogen receptor beta (ER-β), not estrogen receptor alpha (ER-α).
- Why does this matter? Because ER-β is the "regulated" receptor. When isoflavones bind here, they

calm cell growth, balance hormones, and even suppress tumor formation.
- ER-α, by contrast, is the "unregulated" receptor. When overstimulated — often by high estrogen levels in the body or exposure to animal estrogens — ER-α drives uncontrolled growth, fueling cancers like breast and prostate cancer.

In simple terms:

- Isoflavones guide estrogen activity down the regulated beta pathway (protective).
- They reduce overstimulation of the alpha pathway (harmful and unregulated).

That's why populations that eat whole soy foods — tofu, tempeh, miso, edamame — consistently have lower rates of hormone-related cancers.

Soy doesn't fuel cancer. It helps regulate the very receptors that keep cell growth in check.

3. "Beans are poor people's food."

Yes — and that's part of their power. For centuries, beans have been the affordable foundation of survival. They fed soldiers, farmers, families, and entire civilizations. Lentils, chickpeas, peas, and beans were staples from Mesopotamia to Mexico.

Health isn't reserved for the wealthy. Beans prove that life-saving food can be cheap, accessible, and abundant. They don't need branding or billion-dollar marketing campaigns. They just need a pot of water and heat.

What the world calls "peasant food" is really longevity food.

Legumes in Global Traditions

Legumes are not just Blue Zone foods — they are woven into the culinary history of nearly every culture.

- **India:** Lentils (dal) are central to daily meals, often paired with rice or flatbreads.
- **Middle East:** Chickpeas become hummus, falafel, and stews; lentils star in mujaddara.
- **Latin America:** Black beans, pinto beans, and kidney beans anchor rice-and-bean traditions.
- **Mediterranean:** Lentil soups, chickpea salads, and fava beans are ancient staples.
- **Africa:** Cowpeas, black-eyed peas, and pigeon peas nourish millions daily.
- **China & Japan:** Soybeans appear as tofu, tempeh, soy milk, miso, and natto — foods linked to lower cancer rates.

No matter the geography, legumes have been humanity's equalizer food — inexpensive, abundant, versatile, and sustaining.

Beans: The Affordable Medicine

Healthcare costs soar. Supplements and powders flood the market. Yet the most powerful medicine may be sitting in the bulk bin at your grocery store for less than a dollar a pound.

- **One cup of dried beans = pennies per serving.**
- **High nutrient density per calorie.** More protein, fiber, and minerals than most animal products at a fraction of the cost.
- **Shelf stable.** Beans store for months or years, reducing waste and ensuring food security.

For communities battling hunger, beans prevent malnutrition. For families battling obesity, beans restore satiety and balance. For societies battling chronic disease, beans lower costs by reducing the need for drugs.

Beans are proof that health doesn't have to be expensive.

Beans as the Ultimate Equalizer

Think of beans as the **great equalizer of diets.**

- Rich and poor can afford them.
- Every culture can prepare them.
- They are as healing in a Michelin-starred lentil stew as in a simple pot of black beans and rice.

No matter where you live, beans fit in. They adapt to flavors, cuisines, and traditions. And they deliver the same health magic everywhere: strength, satiety, cancer protection, heart health, and longevity.

If there were a single food to unite the world around health, it would be beans.

Stories That Make It Real
David's Heart Health Turnaround

David had battled high cholesterol for years. He ate lean chicken and fish, thinking they were "healthy proteins." But his cholesterol stayed stubbornly high. On a friend's suggestion, he swapped meat for lentils, black beans, and chickpeas. Within six months, his cholesterol plummeted by nearly 50 points. His doctor asked what medication he was on. David smiled and said, "Beans."

Sophia's Cancer Journey

Sophia was diagnosed with early-stage breast cancer. She was terrified, especially after hearing myths about soy "feeding cancer." But after learning the truth — that isoflavones bind to the beta estrogen receptor (regulated and protective) and not the alpha receptor (unregulated and harmful) — she embraced soy. She added tofu, tempeh, and miso soup into her diet. Her energy improved, her treatment side effects were milder, and she felt empowered knowing her food was supporting healing, not working against it.

Marcus's Weight Loss Success

Marcus had struggled with weight for decades. He tried low-carb diets, high-protein plans, and every fad that came along. Nothing lasted. When he switched to a bean-based diet — black bean chili, lentil soup, hummus wraps — something changed. The fiber kept him full, the protein stabilized his blood sugar, and his cravings disappeared. Over 18 months, he lost 70 pounds without feeling deprived. Beans were his turning point.

Elena's Digestive Reset

Elena avoided beans for years because they gave her gas. But her gut health was poor: constipation, bloating, and frequent infections. On her nutritionist's advice, she reintroduced beans slowly, rinsing and cooking them thoroughly. At first, she had mild discomfort, but within weeks, her digestion improved dramatically. The fiber reshaped her microbiome, and she noticed fewer infections and better mood stability. Gas was just part of the adjustment — healing was the long-term result.

These stories share one clear lesson: **legumes don't just nourish — they transform.**

Practical Ways to Eat More Legumes

Making beans part of your daily routine is simple and affordable. Here are some ideas:

1. **Add beans to salads.** Chickpeas, black beans, or kidney beans turn salads into full meals.
2. **Make lentil soup weekly.** It's hearty, inexpensive, and endlessly adaptable.
3. **Snack on roasted chickpeas.** Crunchy, satisfying, and loaded with protein.
4. **Swap beans for meat in tacos, chili, or stews.** Black bean tacos, lentil chili, or chickpea curry are flavorful and filling.
5. **Blend beans into dips.** Hummus, white bean dip, or black bean spread add creaminess without dairy.
6. **Cook in bulk.** Make a large pot of beans on the weekend and use them in multiple dishes during the week.
7. **Experiment with global cuisines.** Indian dal, Mexican frijoles, Middle Eastern falafel, or Japanese miso showcase beans in delicious ways.

Consistency matters more than perfection. Aim for at least one cup daily.

Expanded Key Takeaways

- **Legumes are nutritional powerhouses.** They deliver protein, fiber, minerals, vitamins, and phytochemicals in one package.
- **They are the common thread of longevity.** Every Blue Zone population eats beans daily.
- **They regulate hormones.** Isoflavones in soy bind preferentially to the beta estrogen receptor (ER-β), providing balance and protection instead of overstimulation.
- **They protect against cancer.** Fiber sweeps toxins from the gut, antioxidants neutralize free radicals, and saponins slow tumor growth.
- **They support weight control.** Beans are among the most filling foods on Earth, reducing cravings and balancing blood sugar.
- **They heal the gut.** Bean fiber feeds bacteria that produce SCFAs, which reduce inflammation and support immunity.
- **They are accessible and affordable.** Beans prove that the most powerful medicine is often the cheapest food in the store.

Action Steps

1. **Add beans to one meal today.** Chili, salad, soup, or wrap.
2. **Try a new legume this week.** If you usually eat black beans, try lentils or chickpeas.
3. **Replace one meat meal with beans.** Save money, calories, and improve health.

4. **Aim for one cup daily.** Over time, your microbiome adapts, and benefits multiply.
5. **Explore global bean dishes.** Expand your flavor horizons while building longevity.

Closing Message

Beans may be humble, but they are mighty.

The truth is simple: **if you want to live longer, eat beans — every day.**

In **The P53 Diet & Lifestyle,** I showed how legumes stabilize blood sugar, extend lifespan, and deliver satiety without excess calories. In **Taste Versus Cancer,** I detailed how isoflavones, fiber, and antioxidants in legumes block cancer at the cellular level.

This book keeps the message clear: **beans are the ultimate longevity food.** Affordable, versatile, and protective, they are proof that the path to health doesn't require expensive supplements or complicated diets. It requires opening a bag of lentils, a can of chickpeas, or a pot of black beans.

Longevity doesn't come from mystery superfoods. It comes from the humble legume.

Chapter 10

Nuts & Seeds: Small Packages, Big Power

Nuts and seeds don't look like much. A handful here, a sprinkle there. No bold colors like fruit, no leafy vibrance like vegetables. Yet these tiny foods are among the most nutrient-dense on Earth.

For decades they were dismissed as fattening "snacks." Today, the science is clear: **regular nut and seed eaters live longer, with dramatically lower rates of heart disease, cancer, diabetes, and dementia.**

Small but mighty, nuts and seeds pack concentrated nutrition into portable packages.

Why Nuts and Seeds Heal

Nuts and seeds deliver a combination of nutrients rarely matched by any other food group:

- **Healthy fats:** Omega-3 fatty acids and monounsaturated fats protect the heart, calm inflammation, and nourish the brain.
- **Protein:** Complete amino acid profiles when combined across different seeds and nuts.

- **Fiber:** Supports digestion, lowers cholesterol, and feeds gut bacteria.
- **Minerals:** Magnesium (nerve and muscle health), selenium (DNA protection), zinc (immune and reproductive function), calcium (bones and teeth).
- **Antioxidants:** Vitamin E, lignans, polyphenols, and plant sterols that stabilize free radicals and reduce oxidative stress.

Unlike refined oils or animal fats, nuts and seeds provide fat in the whole-food package — bundled with minerals, protein, antioxidants, and fiber. That synergy is what makes them medicine.

Heart Protection

Cardiovascular disease remains the world's leading killer, but nut and seed eaters enjoy extraordinary protection.

- **LDL cholesterol drops** when nuts replace processed snacks or animal fats. Almonds, walnuts, and pistachios are especially effective.
- **Blood vessel function improves** thanks to arginine, an amino acid that boosts nitric oxide and relaxes arteries.
- **Blood pressure regulation** improves with magnesium- and potassium-rich seeds like pumpkin and flax.
- **Inflammation decreases,** reducing the progression of atherosclerosis.

Large-scale studies consistently show that eating just one handful of nuts per day lowers heart disease risk by 20–30%.

That's more effective than many prescription drugs — without the side effects.

Brain Boost

The brain thrives on the fats and minerals concentrated in nuts and seeds.

- **Walnuts** contain plant-based omega-3s (ALA) that reduce neuroinflammation, support memory, and protect against cognitive decline.
- **Pumpkin seeds** are rich in zinc, crucial for neuro-transmitter function and memory.
- **Flax and chia seeds** provide steady omega-3s that maintain brain cell membranes.
- **Vitamin E** from almonds and sunflower seeds reduces oxidative stress in the brain, slowing dementia progression.

Nut and seed eaters consistently perform better on memory tests, exhibit sharper thinking, and show reduced dementia risk in long-term studies.

The Cancer Connection

Nuts and seeds don't just protect the heart and brain — they also defend against cancer.

- **Flaxseed lignans** act as phytoestrogens that bind to the beta estrogen receptor (regulated and protective), reducing estrogen-driven cancer risk.
- **Selenium in Brazil nuts** repairs DNA, enhances antioxidant defenses, and suppresses tumor initiation.

- **Vitamin E** in almonds, hazelnuts, and sunflower seeds shields cells from oxidative DNA damage.
- **Polyphenols and saponins** in seeds and nuts neutralize free radicals and inhibit cancer cell proliferation.

Population studies confirm that people who regularly consume nuts and seeds have lower rates of breast, prostate, and colon cancers.

Weight and Satiety

Many people avoid nuts because they're calorie-dense. But the evidence tells a different story:

- Nut eaters weigh **less**, not more.
- Why? Nuts are filling, curb cravings, and displace less healthy snacks.
- Not all calories are absorbed. Studies show 10–15% of nut calories are lost through incomplete digestion.

Instead of causing weight gain, nuts promote appetite control and metabolic balance.

Seeds: Nature's Concentrates

Seeds are concentrated nutrition factories.

- **Flax & chia:** Rich in omega-3s, soluble fiber, and lignans that reduce cancer risk.
- **Hemp:** Complete protein with all nine essential amino acids.
- **Pumpkin:** Loaded with magnesium, zinc, and iron for energy and immune function.

- **Sesame:** Packed with calcium, copper, and lignans that balance hormones.
- **Sunflower:** High in vitamin E and selenium, shielding DNA from oxidative damage.

Every tablespoon is like a mini-multivitamin — straight from nature.

How Nuts and Seeds Protect the Heart at the Cellular Level

The heart thrives when arteries stay flexible and blood flows smoothly. Nuts and seeds improve these functions through several biochemical pathways:

1. **LDL Cholesterol Reduction:** Plant sterols in nuts compete with cholesterol for absorption, lowering LDL while leaving HDL (the "good cholesterol") intact.
2. **Nitric Oxide Production:** Arginine in walnuts, pumpkin seeds, and almonds boosts nitric oxide, a compound that dilates blood vessels, lowers blood pressure, and prevents clots.
3. **Antioxidant Defense:** Vitamin E and polyphenols prevent LDL oxidation — the first step in artery-clogging plaque formation.
4. **Anti-Inflammatory Action:** Omega-3s from flax, chia, and walnuts suppress inflammatory cytokines, reducing arterial stiffness.

The result: fewer blockages, lower blood pressure, and improved blood flow. Clinical trials confirm that people who add nuts to their diets reduce cardiovascular events by up to 30%.

Cancer Defense: Why Seeds and Nuts Are Shields

Cancer develops when DNA damage accumulates, cells divide uncontrollably, and immune surveillance fails. Nuts and seeds fight at each stage:

- **DNA Protection:** Selenium from Brazil nuts activates glutathione peroxidase, an enzyme that shields DNA from oxidative damage.
- **Hormone Regulation:** Flaxseed lignans bind preferentially to the beta estrogen receptor (regulated, protective), reducing overstimulation of the alpha receptor (unregulated, harmful). This explains flax's ability to lower breast and prostate cancer risk.
- **Anti-Proliferative Compounds:** Polyphenols and saponins in nuts disrupt signaling pathways that cancer cells use to divide.
- **Apoptosis Promotion:** Certain seed compounds (like ellagic acid in walnuts and flax) encourage damaged cells to self-destruct before turning malignant.

Every handful of nuts or sprinkle of seeds is like flipping genetic switches toward protection instead of promotion.

Nuts, Seeds, and Brain Longevity

Cognitive decline often stems from oxidative stress, inflammation, and poor circulation. Nuts and seeds address all three:

- **Walnuts:** Their ALA omega-3s cross into the brain and integrate into cell membranes, improving neuron function.
- **Pumpkin Seeds:** High zinc levels stabilize neurotransmitter activity, sharpening memory and focus.

- **Almonds & Sunflower Seeds:** Vitamin E reduces oxidative stress that accelerates dementia.
- **Chia & Flax:** Provide precursors for DHA, the omega-3 essential for brain development and memory.

Long-term studies show nut eaters experience slower brain aging and retain better memory into old age. The evidence is so strong that walnuts are often called "food for the brain" — their very shape a reminder of their purpose.

Longevity Cultures and Nuts

Blue Zones — the longest-lived populations — consistently include nuts and seeds:

- **Okinawa, Japan:** Sesame seeds and soybeans are used in sauces, soups, and daily condiments.
- **Ikaria, Greece:** Walnuts and almonds accompany fruits and vegetables, often in honeyed desserts.
- **Sardinia, Italy:** Almonds appear in daily cooking, breads, and celebratory dishes.
- **Nicoya, Costa Rica:** Pumpkin seeds ("pepitas") are staples in sauces and snacks.
- **Loma Linda, California (Adventists):** Nuts are emphasized as daily foods; Adventists who eat nuts regularly live years longer than those who don't.

The pattern is undeniable: where nuts and seeds are daily foods, lifespans stretch.

Myth-Busting Nuts and Seeds
Myth #1: "Nuts make you fat."

The calorie density of nuts makes people nervous. Yet nut eaters consistently weigh less. Why?

- They increase satiety, reducing cravings for junk.
- Up to 15% of nut calories pass through undigested due to their fiber-rich structure.
- Their healthy fats improve insulin sensitivity, reducing fat storage.

The science is clear: nuts don't promote obesity — they prevent it.

Myth #2: "They're just snacks."

Nuts and seeds are not "just" snacks. They are nutritional powerhouses. A handful of almonds or sunflower seeds can rival the nutrient density of a full meal of processed food. Unlike chips or cookies, they heal as they satisfy.

Myth #3: "They're optional."

Nothing could be further from the truth. Nuts and seeds are longevity essentials. Their protective compounds are difficult to replace elsewhere in the diet. Populations that avoid them (or consume very little) consistently show higher rates of chronic disease.

Why Nuts and Seeds Matter Today

In a world of ultra-processed food, nuts and seeds are the antidote. They are:

- Portable and shelf-stable.
- Rich in rare nutrients like selenium and lignans.
- A bridge between ancient survival foods and modern superfoods.

They prove that sometimes the smallest packages carry the biggest protection.

Stories That Make It Real
Michael's Heart Recovery

Michael, 60, had a family history of heart disease. Despite jogging regularly, his cholesterol crept higher each year. Instead of another pill, he decided to try food as medicine. He swapped his afternoon chips for almonds and pistachios, and added ground flaxseed to his morning oatmeal. Within four months, his LDL dropped by 35 points, and his cardiologist called the results "remarkable." Michael now says, "Nuts saved my heart."

Sofia's Menopause Relief

Sofia, 52, struggled with hot flashes and mood swings. Her doctor suggested hormone therapy, but she wanted a natural approach. She began adding flax and chia seeds daily. Within weeks, her symptoms eased. The lignans in flax bound to her beta estrogen receptors (the regulated, protective pathway), helping balance her hormones naturally. She felt calmer, slept better, and regained energy.

Ravi's Brain Boost

Ravi, a graduate student, often complained of brain fog during exams. A mentor suggested walnuts and pumpkin seeds daily. Within a semester, he noticed sharper focus and better memory retention. His study sessions felt more productive, and he credits those simple foods with helping him finish his degree strong.

Elena's Weight Loss Journey

Elena avoided nuts for years, thinking they were "too fattening." Yet she struggled with cravings, binge-eating, and yo-yo dieting. When she began carrying bags of almonds, walnuts, and sunflower seeds as snacks, everything changed. She felt full, satisfied, and gradually stopped craving sweets. Over a year, she lost 40 pounds — not by cutting calories, but by choosing calories that nourished instead of spiked cravings.

These stories show that nuts and seeds aren't luxuries or side snacks. They are tools of healing — working on the heart, brain, hormones, and weight, often when nothing else seems to help.

Practical Ways to Eat More Nuts & Seeds

It doesn't take much to see benefits. A single handful daily is enough to change biomarkers and reduce disease risk. Here's how to make it effortless:

1. **Start Your Day Smart.** Add ground flax or chia to oatmeal, or smoothies.
2. **Snack Wisely.** Keep almonds, walnuts, or sunflower seeds in small containers or bags for portable, filling snacks.
3. **Dress Up Salads.** Sprinkle pumpkin seeds, hemp hearts, or sesame seeds over greens for crunch and nutrition.
4. **Upgrade Dinners.** Use nut-based sauces like cashew cream in place of heavy dressings.
5. **Bake Better.** Replace some flour with almond meal or ground flax in muffins and breads.

6. **Go Global.** Try Mediterranean, Indian sesame chutneys, or Latin pepita sauces. Cultural traditions know how to make nuts and seeds delicious.

The key is **consistency.** One handful occasionally helps, but daily intake makes them true longevity foods.

Expanded Key Takeaways

- **Nuts and seeds = small packages with big power.** They deliver healthy fats, plant protein, minerals, antioxidants, and fiber.
- **They protect the heart.** Lower LDL, relax arteries, and reduce inflammation.
- **They sharpen the brain.** Omega-3s, vitamin E, and zinc support memory and reduce dementia risk.
- **They block cancer pathways.** Lignans, selenium, and polyphenols regulate hormones, repair DNA, and promote apoptosis of abnormal cells.
- **They aid weight control.** High satiety, nutrient density, and partial calorie loss during digestion make nuts anti-obesity foods.
- **They are longevity staples.** Found in every long-lived culture, from Ikaria to Loma Linda.
- **They are daily essentials, not optional extras.** A handful can change health outcomes for decades.

Action Steps

1. **Eat one handful (¼ cup) of nuts daily.** Rotate almonds, walnuts, pistachios, and hazelnuts.

2. **Add flax or chia seeds to meals daily.** One to two tablespoons is enough.
3. **Replace one junk snack with nuts.** Keep them visible and ready.
4. **Try a new seed this week.** Hemp hearts, pumpkin seeds, or sesame may surprise you.
5. **Make nuts and seeds staples, not garnishes.** Build meals around them.

Closing Message

Nuts and seeds may be small, but their impact is massive.

The truth is simple: **a handful a day protects your heart, brain, hormones, and future.**

In *The P53 Diet & Lifestyle*, I emphasized nuts and seeds as daily essentials for long life and chronic disease prevention. In *Taste Versus Cancer,* I documented how flax, walnuts, and Brazil nuts deliver compounds that regulate hormones, block tumor growth, and repair DNA.

This book distills the lesson even further: **don't underestimate the small packages.**

Every almond, walnut, sunflower seed, or spoonful of flax is a dose of concentrated medicine from nature. Taken daily, they don't just extend life — they improve the quality of it.

Big power, small package. That's the gift of nuts and seeds.

Chapter 11

Toxins: Hidden Poisons in Everyday Life

When people hear the word "toxins," they often picture barrels of nuclear waste or smokestacks belching chemicals into the sky. But toxins are not just industrial accidents or distant hazards. They are woven into everyday life.

You don't have to live near a refinery to be poisoned. You just have to:

- Drink tap water with fluoride or aluminum residues.
- Eat processed foods filled with preservatives, dyes, and sweeteners.
- Take pills with synthetic compounds that your body sees as foreign.
- Receive an injection that contains stabilizers or adjuvants that aren't as harmless as advertised.
- Breathe polluted city air.

The body is incredible at detoxification. The liver, kidneys, lungs, gut, and skin are designed to neutralize waste. But modern life overwhelms this natural defense. Instead of clearing a few natural toxins from food or environment, your body is bombarded daily with thousands of chemicals it was never designed to handle.

And when the load exceeds capacity, the result is chronic disease.

Types of Toxins
1. Food Additives

Preservatives like sodium benzoate, dyes like Red 40, and artificial sweeteners may look harmless on a label, but research links them to hyperactivity, allergies, DNA damage, and even cancer. The food industry prizes shelf life — but it's your life that shortens in the process.

2. Pesticides

Sprayed on fruits and vegetables, pesticides seep into every bite. They disrupt hormones, damage nerve function, and accumulate in fat tissue. Even low levels have been tied to higher risks of cancer and neurological decline.

3. Dyes

Brightly colored candies, cereals, and sodas often contain petroleum-based dyes. Studies link these to ADHD, mood disturbances, and liver toxicity. A child's tantrum may not be "bad behavior" — it may be a reaction to Red 40 or Yellow 5.

4. Vaccines & Drugs

These are not without baggage. Many vaccines contain aluminum salts as adjuvants. Aluminum is a known neurotoxin that accumulates in brain and bone tissue. Some also contain preservatives that challenge the liver. Drugs — from antibiotics to antidepressants — may mask symptoms, but they almost always come with side effects and nutrient depletion. The "cure" can quietly drain the body's reserves, leaving it weaker long term.

5. Smoking

One of the most direct toxins, cigarettes deliver arsenic, cadmium, formaldehyde, and thousands of compounds that scar lungs, stiffen arteries, and mutate DNA.

6. Alcohol

The most socially accepted toxin, alcohol is a liver-damaging carcinogen. Even small amounts raise risks of breast, colon, and liver cancers. It isn't "just a drink." It's a cellular disruptor.

Aluminum and Fluoride: Hidden Poisons

Aluminum is everywhere — cookware, foil, deodorants, antacids, and vaccine adjuvants. Once in the body, it doesn't belong. It crosses the blood-brain barrier, accumulating in neural tissue. Chronic exposure is linked to Alzheimer's, Parkinson's, and impaired bone health. The body has no real mechanism to detoxify heavy metals like aluminum once they build up.

Fluoride is another silent toxin. Promoted as a dental aid, it is added to tap water in many regions. But fluoride is a neurotoxin in high doses, and even "safe levels" have been tied to lower IQ in children, endocrine disruption, and skeletal fluorosis. Ironically, while promoted to "strengthen teeth," excess fluoride can weaken them, causing mottling and brittleness.

Pills as Toxins

Pharmaceutical drugs are often seen as modern miracles. But the body does not recognize them as natural compounds. Each pill is a xenobiotic — a foreign chemical.

- **Statins** deplete coenzyme Q10, starving the heart of fuel.
- **Diuretics** deplete potassium and magnesium, leading to cramps and arrhythmias.

- **Antacids** block stomach acid, interfering with nutrient absorption.
- **Antibiotics** wipe out gut flora, leaving the immune system vulnerable, and have been shown to grow cancer cells.

Drugs may suppress a symptom, but they almost always create nutrient debt — weakening the very systems they aim to support.

Sodium Benzoate + Citric Acid = Benzene

Few people realize that the preservatives in their soda can combine into something far worse.

- **Sodium benzoate** (a preservative)
- **Citric acid** (common in drinks and candies)

When combined under certain conditions (heat, light, time), they form benzene — a known carcinogen linked to leukemia and other blood cancers.

This isn't conspiracy theory — it has been documented by the FDA and independent labs. Some sodas tested in the past contained benzene at levels far above safety standards. The food industry quietly reformulated many products, but sodium benzoate and citric acid still appear together on labels today.

Every sip is a gamble.

The Body's Defense System

The human body is brilliant. It comes equipped with a sophisticated detoxification network designed to neutralize and excrete harmful substances.

- **The Liver** is the body's chemical filter. It transforms fat-soluble toxins into water-soluble compounds that can be excreted. Phase I and Phase II detox pathways depend on nutrients like B vitamins, magnesium, glutathione, and sulfur compounds from cruciferous vegetables.
- **The Kidneys** filter blood, removing waste and balancing minerals. But heavy metals like aluminum and fluoride can strain them and accumulate over time.
- **The Lungs** expel volatile chemicals, carbon dioxide, and airborne toxins. But constant exposure to pollution or cigarette smoke overwhelms their protective linings.
- **The Gut** is both barrier and eliminator. Fiber binds toxins for removal. But when gut flora are destroyed by antibiotics or poor diet, this defense collapses.
- **The Skin** sweats out toxins. Yet lotions, deodorants, and cosmetics often deliver a daily dose of chemicals that bypass filtration entirely.

The system works — but only within limits. When nutrient reserves are low, detox stalls. When the load is constant, the liver and kidneys never catch up. And when hidden toxins slip past, they build up silently in tissues — brain, fat, bones — waiting years before symptoms appear.

The Illusion of Moderation

You've heard the phrase: "Everything in moderation." It's the modern mantra to justify indulgence. A little alcohol, a few cigarettes, an occasional soda — what harm could it do?

Here's the truth: **a little poison is still poison.**

- Would you drink "just a little" arsenic?

- Inject "just a little" mercury?
- Feed your child "just a little" lead paint dust?

Of course not. Yet the same logic is used to normalize alcohol, fluoride, aluminum, or benzene-forming preservatives. These substances have no nutritional value and carry risk at any dose. The idea of moderation is a marketing shield, not a health truth.

Even when single doses are small, the danger is in accumulation. One soda won't cause cancer — but 30 years of sodas may. One aluminum-laced injection won't cause dementia — but decades of aluminum exposure in cookware, deodorants, and adjuvants adds up. The human body is remarkable, but it is not invincible.

How Toxins Damage the Terrain

Most people think of disease as an external invasion — a germ, a gene, bad luck. But toxins shape the terrain inside the body, making it fertile ground for disease.

- **DNA Damage:** Carcinogens like benzene and pesticides attack DNA, creating mutations that lead to cancer.
- **Oxidative Stress:** Aluminum, fluoride, and heavy metals generate free radicals that damage proteins, fats, and cell membranes.
- **Hormone Disruption:** Preservatives, dyes, and pesticides act like endocrine mimics, confusing estrogen, testosterone, and thyroid hormones.
- **Immune Suppression:** Constant toxin exposure exhausts immune cells, leaving the body unable to respond to genuine threats like infections or rogue cancer cells.

· **Nutrient Drain:** Pharmaceuticals, alcohol, and additives burn through vitamins and minerals, creating deficiencies that further weaken detox capacity.

This is why two people exposed to the same germ have different outcomes. The germ is the spark. The terrain — strengthened or weakened by toxins — determines whether there's a fire.

Stories That Make It Real
Anna's Migraines
Anna had lived with crippling migraines for a decade. Doctors prescribed pill after pill, each bringing side effects and little relief. Finally, she overhauled her diet, cutting processed foods with dyes, sodium benzoate, and aspartame. Within weeks, the migraines disappeared. Her "mystery illness" wasn't a lack of pills. It was toxins.

Robert's Fatigue
Robert, 47, felt exhausted every day. He blamed aging. But after quitting alcohol and processed meats, his energy soared. His liver enzymes normalized, and he lost 20 pounds. The problem wasn't age — it was toxic load.

Lisa's Child
Lisa's young son struggled with hyperactivity and mood swings. Teachers suggested medication. Instead, Lisa cut soda, candy, and cereals with artificial dyes. Within a month, his behavior improved dramatically. His brain wasn't broken — it was overstimulated by chemical additives.

These stories show what research confirms: when you remove toxins, the body heals. It doesn't need a detox kit, a fad cleanse, or another prescription. It needs removal of poison and restoration of fuel.

More Stories That Make It Real
Evelyn's Autoimmune Battle

Evelyn, 38, was diagnosed with an autoimmune thyroid condition. She was exhausted, anxious, and losing hair. Doctors offered lifelong medication. Instead, she started by removing fluoride toothpaste, aluminum-based deodorants, and heavily processed snacks with preservatives. She switched to filtered water, plant-rich meals, and natural body care. Six months later, her antibody levels dropped, her hair grew thicker, and her energy returned. Her immune system wasn't attacking randomly — it was reacting to daily toxins.

James's Liver Wake-Up Call

James, a social drinker, thought his nightly glass of wine was "healthy" thanks to moderation myths. But bloodwork revealed elevated liver enzymes. His doctor warned of fatty liver disease. James quit alcohol, ditched processed meats, and began eating cruciferous vegetables daily. Within months, his liver tests normalized. His turnaround proved that the liver isn't weak — it's simply overwhelmed by toxins until you give it relief.

Monica's Child and Learning Struggles

Monica's 9-year-old daughter struggled in school with attention and focus. Teachers hinted at ADHD medication. Instead, Monica pulled foods with sodium benzoate and citric acid from her diet — no more sodas or processed snacks. Within weeks, her daughter's focus improved dramatically. She wasn't broken. She was reacting to benzene-forming additives that her growing body couldn't handle.

These examples reinforce a truth: toxins are not abstract. They impact real lives, every day.

Practical Strategies to Reduce Toxin Exposure

You can't avoid every toxin, but you can drastically reduce your load. Each small change lightens the burden on your body's detox system.

Food Choices

- **Read labels.** If you see sodium benzoate, citric acid, Red 40, Yellow 5, or aspartame, put it back.
- **Choose organic when possible.** Especially for high-residue produce like strawberries, spinach, apples, and grapes.
- **Ditch processed meats.** Bacon, hot dogs, and deli meats often contain nitrates, preservatives, and toxic by-products.
- **Favor whole plants.** Fruits, vegetables, legumes, nuts, and seeds supply fiber, antioxidants, and nutrients that neutralize toxins.

Water & Beverages

- **Filter tap water.** Choose filters that remove fluoride, chlorine, and heavy metals.
- **Avoid sodas and energy drinks.** Especially those with sodium benzoate and citric acid.
- **Drink plenty of clean water.** Hydration supports kidney detox.

Home & Body

- **Switch deodorants.** Avoid aluminum-based antiperspirants.
- **Choose natural cleaners.** Vinegar, baking soda, and plant-based formulas over chemical sprays.
- **Avoid nonstick pans.** Teflon releases toxic fumes. Use stainless steel or cast iron instead.
- **Limit plastics.** BPA and phthalates leach into food. Use glass, stainless steel, or ceramic.

Lifestyle

- **Quit alcohol and smoking completely.** No "moderation."
- **Sweat it out.** Exercise and sauna use promote detox through skin.
- **Support your gut.** Eat high-fiber foods and fermented plants to maintain strong microbiota.
- **Prioritize sleep.** The brain detoxifies most effectively during deep sleep.

Expanded Key Takeaways

- **Toxins are everywhere.** They hide in food, water, air, products, and even pills.
- **The body can detoxify,** but only when supported by nutrients and not overwhelmed.
- **Aluminum and fluoride** disrupt the brain, bones, and immune system.
- **Sodium benzoate + citric acid can create benzene,** a known carcinogen.

- **Pharmaceutical drugs act as toxins,** often depleting nutrients and harming long-term health.
- **Moderation is a myth.** Small doses of poison accumulate over time.
- **Removing toxins heals.** Migraines, fatigue, autoimmune conditions, and learning struggles often improve when toxic load decreases.
- **Plants are the ultimate defense.** Crucifers, garlic, onions, cilantro, and colorful vegetables power detox pathways daily.

Action Steps

1. **Audit your kitchen.** Remove products with dyes, sodium benzoate, citric acid, and artificial sweeteners.
2. **Switch your water source.** Filtered water is non-negotiable.
3. **Detox your home.** Replace aluminum deodorants, nonstick pans, and chemical cleaners.
4. **Add detoxifying plants.** Cruciferous vegetables, garlic, turmeric, and leafy greens daily.
5. **Go alcohol- and smoke-free.** Not "less." Zero.

Closing Message

Toxins are the silent thieves of health. They don't strike like lightning — they erode like acid. A little here, a little there, until the terrain is weak, immunity falters, and disease takes hold.

But here's the good news: **you are not powerless.** Every plant-based choice strengthens your defenses. Every toxin you avoid lightens the load. Every nutrient-dense bite arms your detox system with what it needs.

In **The P53 Diet & Lifestyle,** I showed how toxins weaken the terrain, making the body more vulnerable to cancer and chronic disease. In my book **How You Are Being Poisoned,** I detailed how drugs silently strip nutrients, creating hidden deficiencies that look like mystery illnesses.

This book keeps it simple: **toxins are everywhere, but so are solutions.** They are silent invaders. Plants are your shield.

Chapter 12

Food Labels: Decoding the Lies

Walk down any grocery store aisle and you'll be greeted with bright labels shouting:

- "All Natural"
- "Low Fat"
- "Heart Healthy"
- "Made with Whole Grains"
- "Light"
- "Sugar-Free"

It all sounds good, doesn't it? That's the point. Food companies hire psychologists, designers, and chemists to craft words and images that trigger trust and craving. Labels are not nutrition guides. They are marketing weapons.

The purpose of a label is not to protect your health. It's to protect the company's profit.

How Labels Lie
1. Serving Sizes
The easiest trick in the book. Serving sizes are deliberately tiny to make numbers look harmless. A soda bottle may say "100

calories per serving" — but the bottle is 2.5 servings. Who drinks half a bottle and puts it back? The same goes for chips, cookies, and cereals. Labels shrink serving sizes until poisons look like snacks.

2. "All Natural"

Sounds wholesome. Legally meaningless. High-fructose corn syrup, preservatives, and chemical dyes can all hide under the "natural" umbrella. Arsenic is natural. So is mercury. "Natural" is a word designed to disarm suspicion.

3. "Low Fat"

This often means high sugar. When the fat is removed, flavor is lost — so companies add sugar, corn syrup, or artificial sweeteners. The result? Worse for your metabolism than the original.

4. "Sugar-Free"

Too good to be true? It is. "Sugar-free" products often use aspartame, sucralose, or acesulfame potassium — artificial sweeteners tied to gut damage, headaches, mood disorders, and insulin resistance.

5. "Made with Whole Grains"

Translation: mostly refined flour with a sprinkle of whole wheat for marketing. It's like putting a drop of orange juice in soda and calling it "made with fruit."

6. "Organic Junk"

Organic cookies are still cookies. Organic sugar is still sugar. "Organic" prevents pesticide residues, but it doesn't change the reality of high-calorie, low-nutrient junk food.

Ingredients Don't Lie

The front of the box is advertising. The back of the box is the truth. The ingredient list reveals the real story.

Rules of thumb:

- **Shorter is better.** Five ingredients beat twenty.
- **Recognizable words are better.** If you wouldn't stock it in your kitchen, why eat it?
- **Whole foods first.** If sugar, oil, or chemicals dominate the top three ingredients, put it back.

If the list reads like a chemistry experiment — it's not food.

The Chemistry of "Sodium ..."

One of the biggest red flags on labels is anything that starts with sodium. It's not just about salt (sodium chloride). It's about industrial sodium compounds slipped into food for preservation, texture, or shelf life. Many of these carry serious health risks.

- **Sodium nitrate / sodium nitrite** – Used in processed meats. In the body, they can form nitrosamines, potent carcinogens linked to colon and stomach cancer.
- **Sodium benzoate** – A preservative. Harmless until combined with citric acid or ascorbic acid (vitamin C), where it can form **benzene**, a carcinogen. Linked to hyperactivity in children and mitochondrial damage.
- **Sodium phosphate** – Added to processed cheese, lunch meats, and baked goods. Excess phosphate stresses the kidneys, weakens bones, and accelerates aging.
- **Sodium sulfite** – Preserves dried fruits and wine. Can trigger asthma attacks, headaches, and allergic reactions.
- **Sodium lauryl sulfate (SLS)** – Found in toothpaste and processed foods. Irritates gut lining and damages beneficial bacteria.

These compounds don't nourish. They manipulate texture, extend shelf life, and fake freshness. But inside the body, they corrode health.

Whenever you see "sodium ..." on a label, treat it as a red flag.

Why Labels Exist

Most people assume labels are there to protect consumers. Wrong. Labels were designed to protect companies from lawsuits. As long as the numbers are technically correct — even if they're misleading — the company is safe.

- Serving sizes can be absurdly small.
- Chemical names can be hidden under umbrella terms like "flavoring."
- Marketing terms like "natural" or "light" have no strict definition.

The label system is not about transparency. It's about liability.

The Chemistry of Additives

When you flip a package over, you may not recognize half the ingredients. That's no accident. Labels are written in chemistry-speak — a deliberate language barrier. The more confusing it looks, the less likely you are to question it.

Here are some of the biggest offenders:

1. Artificial Dyes

- *Red 40, Yellow 5, Blue 1* — petroleum-based colorants linked to ADHD, mood swings, and allergies.
- These dyes don't nourish. They're used to trick the eye — to make gray cereal look golden, or candy look like fruit.

· Europe has forced warning labels on some dyes. The U.S. still allows them in children's foods.

2. Artificial Sweeteners

· *Aspartame, Sucralose, Acesulfame K* — all approved as "safe." Yet studies show they harm gut bacteria, disrupt insulin response, and can even trigger headaches or mood changes.
· These aren't food. They're lab-engineered sugar imposters.

3. Preservatives

· *BHA (butylated hydroxyanisole), BHT (butylated hydroxytoluene)* — synthetic antioxidants used to keep fats from spoiling. Classified as possible carcinogens.
· *Propyl gallate* — another antioxidant preservative linked to stomach and liver issues.
· *TBHQ (tertiary butylhydroquinone)* — used in crackers, chips, and frozen foods. Even small amounts cause nausea and DNA damage in lab studies.

These chemicals exist to make food last on shelves — not to make you last longer.

How Labels Are Designed to Confuse
Food companies know the rules — and they know how to bend them.

· **Umbrella terms** like "natural flavors" or "spices" can legally hide dozens of lab-engineered compounds.

- **Splitting sugar** into multiple forms — cane sugar, brown rice syrup, maltodextrin, fructose — so "sugar" doesn't appear first on the list.
- **Serving size games** — slicing a package into unrealistic portions so the numbers look harmless.
- **Health halo phrases** — "cholesterol-free" slapped on foods that never had cholesterol anyway.

The result? Shoppers believe they're making smart choices when they're just buying the same junk in a different box.

The "Sodium ..." Family of Hidden Toxins

Let's dig deeper into why anything that starts with "sodium" should make you stop. These compounds are not table salt. They are industrial chemicals added for manipulation, not nourishment.

- **Sodium Nitrate/Nitrite** — Processed meats (bacon, hot dogs, deli slices). They form nitrosamines in the stomach, potent carcinogens directly tied to colon cancer.
- **Sodium Benzoate** — Preservative in sodas, salad dressings, and condiments. When combined with citric acid or vitamin C, it forms **benzene** — a cancer-causing chemical once used in gasoline.
- **Sodium Phosphate** — Found in "whipped" dairy products, baked goods, and processed meats. It disrupts phosphate balance, stressing kidneys and bones.

· **Sodium Sulfite** — Preservative in dried fruit and wine. Triggers asthma attacks, skin rashes, and headaches.
· **Sodium Lauryl Sulfate (SLS)** — Common in toothpaste and even some processed foods. Harsh on the gut lining and microbiome.

Every one of these exists for the convenience of companies, not for the health of humans.

When you see "sodium ..." on a label, ask: ***Do I want a lab experiment in my body?***

Stories That Make It Real
Janet's "Healthy" Lunch Meat

Janet switched to turkey slices labeled "lean and heart healthy." She ate them daily, proud of her choice. But she didn't notice "sodium nitrite" on the back. Within years, she developed pre-cancerous colon polyps. When she learned about nitrosamines, she dropped processed meats for beans and lentils. Her digestive health improved — and so did her peace of mind.

Carlos's Sports Drink

Carlos grabbed neon-colored sports drinks after workouts, thinking they replaced electrolytes. The front label promised "recovery hydration." The back showed sodium benzoate and Yellow 5. His daily "recovery" was actually daily benzene risk and chemical dyes. Once he swapped for water with lemon and chia seeds, his headaches stopped.

Maya's "Low Fat" Yogurt

Maya ate "low fat" yogurt every morning. The label highlighted "probiotics" and "made with whole grains." The truth: it contained more sugar than a candy bar, plus sodium phosphate to thicken it. On top of that, the dairy itself carried baggage — saturated fat, hormones, and inflammatory proteins that strained her digestion. Her blood sugar spikes explained her mid-morning crashes, while the dairy left her feeling bloated and sluggish. When she replaced it with plain oats, fruit, and flaxseed, her digestion improved and her energy stabilized.

These aren't rare mistakes. They're the rule. Labels are crafted to mislead.

Why Chemistry Matters

Many people shrug at labels. "It's just a little preservative." "It's approved as safe."

But here's the truth: the dose is cumulative.

- One soda with sodium benzoate might not hurt.
- But 20 years of sodas create an internal chemical storm.
- One slice of bacon won't cause cancer.
- But years of nitrite exposure create fertile ground for disease.

Chemistry doesn't care about marketing. Molecules do what they do. And inside your body, they become **slow poisons.**

More Stories That Make It Real
Ethan's "Sugar-Free" Snacks

Ethan, a diabetic, trusted "sugar-free" cookies to be safe. The label showed zero sugar, but hidden inside were aspartame and maltodextrin. His blood sugar still spiked, and he developed constant digestive distress. Only after ditching "sugar-free" products and returning to whole fruits did his energy and blood sugar stabilize.

Samantha's "All Natural" Juice

Samantha bought juice labeled "all natural, no added sugar." But the fine print revealed it was reconstituted from concentrate, with "natural flavors" added to boost sweetness. Drinking it daily packed as much sugar as soda. Her "healthy juice habit" led to weight gain and fatigue. She switched to eating whole oranges and never looked back.

Mark's "Organic" Chips

Mark was proud to buy organic tortilla chips, convinced they were guilt-free. But the label showed organic sunflower oil, sodium phosphate, and natural flavors. They were still fried, salty, and calorie-dense. Organic didn't mean harmless. Once he replaced them with homemade bean-and-veggie wraps, his weight dropped and cravings eased.

A Step-by-Step Method for Decoding Labels

When you can't avoid packaged food, use these steps to protect yourself:

1. **Ignore the Front.** Marketing terms like "natural," "low fat," or "organic" are designed to distract. Flip it over.
2. **Check Serving Size.** Ask yourself: is this realistic? If a "bag" is listed as 3 servings, know the numbers are diluted.
3. **Scan for "Sodium ..." Compounds.** Sodium nitrate, benzoate, phosphate, sulfite — each one is a red flag. If you see it, put it back.

4. **Look for Sugar Tricks.** If sugar hides under multiple names (maltodextrin, cane juice, syrup, fructose), know it's engineered deception.
5. **Watch for Artificial Additives.** Red 40, Yellow 5, aspartame, sucralose, BHA, BHT, TBHQ — these are industrial chemicals, not food.
6. **Count Ingredients.** Shorter lists are safer. Five whole-food ingredients beat twenty chemicals.
7. **Prioritize Whole Foods.** If the first three ingredients aren't recognizable plants, it's not nourishing.

The faster you scan, the clearer the truth becomes: **most labels hide poison under fancy packaging.**

Expanded Key Takeaways

- **Labels are marketing tools, not health guides.**
- **Serving sizes are manipulated.** Numbers shrink while portions don't.
- **"All Natural" means nothing.** Poison can be natural.
- **"Low Fat" usually means high sugar.**
- **"Sugar-Free" hides chemical imposters.**
- **"Made with Whole Grains" is a sprinkle of truth in a loaf of lies.**
- **"Organic" doesn't erase junk.** Organic sugar is still sugar.
- **Sodium compounds are red flags.** Nitrate, benzoate, phosphate, sulfite — all harmful.
- **Ingredient lists tell the truth.** Short, simple, recognizable = safe.
- **The best food has no label at all.** Apples, beans, spinach, carrots don't need marketing.

Action Steps

1. **Audit your pantry.** Pull one packaged food, flip it over, and read the ingredients aloud. Can you pronounce them? Do they sound like food?
2. **Ditch the sodium compounds.** If it starts with "sodium ..." and it isn't salt, cut it out.
3. **Replace one packaged snack with real food.** Fruit, raw nuts, or homemade beans.
4. **Shop the perimeter.** Produce, bulk bins, and fresh foods are safer than aisles of boxes.
5. **Make it a habit.** Every time you shop, practice scanning labels — soon it will take seconds to spot deception.

Closing Message

Food labels are a legal mask. The front sells health. The back hides poison.

The truth is simple: **real food doesn't need labels.** No apple brags it's "low fat." No lentil needs a "made with whole grains" sticker. No head of broccoli is "all natural."

In **The P53 Diet & Lifestyle**, I explained how labels are used to disguise toxins and manipulate perception. In **Taste Versus Cancer**, I showed how food additives create terrain for disease. In my book **How You Are Being Poisoned** I cover this and so much more.

This book distills the message: **labels lie. Ingredients tell the truth.** And the ultimate truth is this: the healthiest foods come without labels at all.

Chapter 13

Ailments: Listening to the Body's Signals

Most people treat ailments as annoyances to get rid of:

- Headache? Take a painkiller.
- Heartburn? Pop an antacid.
- Fatigue? Grab caffeine.
- High blood pressure? Swallow a pill.
- High cholesterol? Take a statin.

We've been trained to silence symptoms instead of asking what they mean.

But here's the truth: **symptoms are signals.** They are the body's language, designed to communicate imbalance. A headache isn't random. Fatigue isn't weakness. High cholesterol isn't an accident. They're messages.

Ignore the whispers, and the body speaks louder. Suppress the signals, and the root fire keeps burning.

How Ailments Work
Every symptom has a story behind it.

- **Headaches** may point to dehydration, magnesium deficiency, excess sodium, or toxic overload.
- **Fatigue** could signal anemia, thyroid imbalance, sleep disruption, nutrient deficiency, or chronic inflammation.
- **Digestive issues** often reveal gut imbalance, food intolerances, or overprocessed diets.
- **Skin problems** reflect the liver's struggle, food sensitivities, or toxin exposure.
- **Joint pain** may stem from inflammation caused by excess animal protein, dairy, or oils.

The key is not to numb the symptom but to ask: ***why is this happening?***

The Pill Trap

Modern medicine excels at symptom suppression. Pills are quick, easy, and profitable. But pills don't heal. They mute.

- **Antacids** relieve heartburn but block stomach acid, impairing nutrient absorption.
- **Painkillers** ease headaches but damage the liver or gut over time.
- **Allergy medications** mask reactions while the immune system grows weaker.
- **Sleep aids** force rest but create dependence and brain fog.

Even worse, drugs often create side effects that become new ailments. A pill for digestion leads to nutrient deficiency. A pill for blood pressure causes fatigue. A statin for cholesterol causes muscle pain — and the cycle continues.

The Blood Pressure Pill Problem

High blood pressure (hypertension) is one of the most common diagnoses in the world. The reflex solution? Pills.

But blood pressure medications don't fix the cause. They tinker with the body's plumbing while leaving the pressure behind untouched. Worse, they create new problems:

- **Diuretics** flush out fluid, but also drain potassium and magnesium — leaving muscles cramping and the heart vulnerable.
- **Beta-blockers** lower heart rate, but sap energy, blunt mood, and reduce exercise capacity.
- **ACE inhibitors** disrupt hormonal balance, often causing chronic cough, dizziness, or kidney strain.

The body never had a "pill deficiency." Hypertension often stems from excess sodium, low potassium, poor circulation, obesity, stress, and toxic diet. A plant-based diet, exercise, and stress reduction fix the root. Pills only patch the symptom.

The LDL-Lowering Statin Trap

High cholesterol is another red flag — a signal that the diet and terrain are out of balance. Statins are handed out like candy to suppress LDL numbers. But the damage runs deep:

- **Statins deplete Coenzyme Q10 (CoQ10),** a critical compound for energy production in the heart and muscles. Depletion weakens the very organ they're supposed to protect.
- They cause muscle pain and weakness, sometimes permanent.
- They can trigger cognitive issues, including memory loss and confusion.

- They may impair blood sugar control, raising diabetes risk.

Statins lower numbers on paper but don't resolve the true cause: excess animal fat, processed foods, and lack of fiber. Only plants lower LDL naturally by providing soluble fiber, antioxidants, and phytosterols — without side effects.

Listening Instead of Silencing

What if, instead of fighting ailments, we listened?

- A headache might mean drink more water, ease stress, or add magnesium-rich greens.
- Fatigue might mean adjust sleep, check iron, and improve diet.
- Heartburn might mean cut dairy, oils, and processed foods.
- High blood pressure might mean eat more potassium-rich plants (bananas, beans, spinach) and reduce sodium.
- High cholesterol might mean replace meat and cheese with beans, oats, and nuts.

Symptoms don't mean the body is failing. They mean the body is working — sending alarms so you can respond.

Pills and Nutrient Depletion

Every drug works by interfering with normal biochemistry. That interference doesn't just block symptoms — it often robs the body of vital nutrients.

- **Diuretics (blood pressure pills):** Flush water and electrolytes, but also strip magnesium, potassium, zinc, and B vitamins. Deficiencies lead to muscle cramps, arrhythmias, depression, and fatigue.

- **Statins (LDL-lowering pills):** Block cholesterol synthesis but also block production of **CoQ10,** the spark plug of mitochondria. Without CoQ10, energy falters and the heart itself weakens.
- **Antacids and PPIs:** Neutralize acid, but also block absorption of iron, calcium, magnesium, and B12. The result? Anemia, brittle bones, neurological decline.
- **Antibiotics:** Destroy pathogens but also wipe out beneficial gut flora. Without gut flora, digestion falters, immunity collapses, and mood disorders increase.
- **Painkillers (NSAIDs):** Suppress inflammation, but also damage the stomach lining, increasing risk of ulcers and gut bleeding.

Each pill is like solving a leaky pipe by hammering the alarm — the water still rises, and now the alarm is broken.

Ailments and the Terrain

Terrain theory says disease arises not from invaders but from the internal environment. Ailments are the early warnings that the terrain is faltering.

- High blood pressure? The blood vessels are inflamed, stiffened by cholesterol, sodium, and oxidative stress.
- High cholesterol? The liver is overloaded with animal fat, dairy proteins, and lack of soluble fiber.
- Heartburn? The digestive terrain is inflamed by oils, processed food, and animal products.
- Skin rashes? The body is detoxing through the skin because the liver is overworked.

· Fatigue? The terrain is nutrient-depleted, toxin-heavy, or chronically inflamed.

Suppressing these signals with pills does not heal the terrain — it hides the damage until it worsens.

Stories That Make It Real
David's Blood Pressure Cycle

David, 55, was prescribed diuretics for high blood pressure. At first, numbers improved. But soon he developed muscle cramps and constant fatigue. His doctor prescribed magnesium supplements — then another pill for sleep. Still, nothing solved the cause. Finally, David shifted to a plant-based diet rich in beans, greens, and potassium. Within six months, his blood pressure normalized without drugs. His terrain healed — and so did his energy.

Angela's Statin Struggle

Angela, 62, was put on statins for "high LDL." Within months, she developed muscle aches so severe she couldn't walk her dog. Her doctor suggested another drug for pain. Instead, she read about soluble fiber, oats, beans, and walnuts. She adopted a plant-based lifestyle, dropped her LDL naturally, and regained her mobility. She laughs now: "I didn't need a pill. I needed plants."

Carlos and the Antacid Trap

Carlos suffered from heartburn. Antacids became his daily crutch. Years later, he was diagnosed with osteoporosis and anemia. The connection? Antacids had blocked his calcium, magnesium, and iron absorption for years. When he cut processed oils, fried foods, and dairy — and added vegetables, beans, and whole grains — his heartburn vanished. He tossed the pills for good.

Lena's Fatigue Mystery

Lena, 40, battled daily fatigue. Bloodwork showed "normal" results, so doctors offered antidepressants. Instead, she tracked her diet and realized most meals were processed snacks and energy drinks. She replaced them with plant-based meals — quinoa, lentils, fruit, greens — and within weeks, her fatigue lifted. She wasn't "depressed." She was malnourished.

Robert's "Normal" Aging

Robert, 67, believed fatigue and joint pain were "just aging." His doctor added blood pressure pills, then cholesterol pills. Soon he was on six prescriptions. Still, he felt worse. His daughter encouraged him to try plant-based eating. Within a year, he was off four of his six drugs, his joints stopped aching, and he hiked again with his grandchildren. Aging wasn't the problem. Pills were.

Sophia's Skin Struggles

Sophia, 29, fought constant acne. Dermatologists prescribed creams, antibiotics, and hormones. Nothing solved it. When she removed dairy and processed oils from her diet, her skin cleared within months. The symptom wasn't random — it was her body saying, ***"Stop feeding me toxins."***

Greg's Headaches

Greg popped painkillers daily for headaches. Scans showed nothing serious, so doctors dismissed it as "stress." Finally, a nutritionist suggested hydration and magnesium-rich foods like pumpkin seeds, spinach, and beans. Within weeks, his headaches vanished. The problem wasn't in his head. It was in his diet.

Elena's High Blood Pressure

Elena, 51, relied on medication for hypertension. She believed she'd be on it for life. But the side effects — fatigue, dizziness — kept piling up. She joined a plant-based support group, reduced sodium, added beans and greens, and walked daily. Within nine months, she was pill-free with normal blood pressure. Her body wasn't broken. It was waiting for nourishment.

A Step-by-Step Approach to Listening

1. **Pause Before Popping a Pill.** The next time a symptom arises, resist the reflex to silence it. Ask: *what is my body telling me?*
2. **Track Symptoms.** Keep a simple journal. Patterns often reveal food triggers, sleep problems, or stress links.
3. **Check Lifestyle Factors.**
   - Am I hydrated?
   - Am I sleeping enough?
   - Am I overloaded with stress?
   - Am I eating real food or processed junk?
4. **Adjust Food First.** Remove dairy, oils, excess sodium, and processed foods. Add greens, beans, whole grains, nuts, seeds, and fruit.
5. **Move and Rest.** Gentle activity and deep rest reset systems more effectively than pills.
6. **Seek Root Causes, Not Quick Fixes.** If medication is prescribed, ask: *what is this covering up?* Then look deeper.

Your body is not attacking you. It's guiding you — if you're willing to listen.

Expanded Key Takeaways

- **Symptoms are signals, not mistakes.** They are your body's language.
- **Pills silence alarms but don't solve causes.** Blood pressure pills, statins, antacids, and painkillers all create new problems.
- **Every ailment points to imbalance.** Diet, toxins, stress, and deficiencies are the real culprits.
- **Listening prevents disease.** Responding early to signals avoids the spiral of chronic illness.
- **Plant-based living heals terrain.** Whole foods, water, rest, and movement resolve the cause, not just the symptom.

Action Steps

1. **Keep a symptom journal for one month.** Record headaches, fatigue, digestion, skin, mood. Look for patterns.
2. **Replace one pill with a plant-based solution.** Try magnesium-rich seeds for cramps, water for headaches, or greens for blood pressure.

3. **Audit your prescriptions.** Ask your doctor what nutrients they deplete — then replace those with food.

4. **Practice curiosity.** When a symptom arises, pause. Instead of asking *"How do I stop this?"* ask *"What is this teaching me?"*

Closing Message

Your body is not against you. It's for you. Every ache, rash, spike, or dip is communication — not failure. Pills may silence the voice, but they never heal the cause.

The truth is simple: **ailments are messages. Listen before they scream.**

In **The P53 Diet & Lifestyle**, I showed how ignoring early signals leads to chronic disease. In my work on pharmaceuticals, I detailed how pills mask problems while depleting the very nutrients needed for healing.

This book keeps it clear: **your body speaks the language of symptoms. Learn to listen. Choose plants, rest, and balance — not pills.**

Chapter 14

Cancers: When the Body's Alarms Are Ignored

A sk most people why cancer happens, and you'll hear three answers:

- "It's bad luck."
- "It's in my genes."
- "It just happens."

But cancer isn't random. Cancer is not a lightning strike from the sky. It is a **terrain disease.**

Genes may load the gun, but lifestyle pulls the trigger. And here's the good news: you can choose not to pull it.

Cancer begins when cells are damaged and fail to repair themselves. Normally, the immune system patrols like a security guard, spotting these rogue cells and eliminating them. But when the **terrain is weak** — starved of nutrients, overloaded with toxins, inflamed by poor diet — cancer slips through the cracks. Those rogue cells multiply, recruit blood vessels, and grow into tumors.

Cancer is not fate. It's fuel plus terrain.

What Cancer Really Is

At its core, cancer is the breakdown of three protective systems:

1. **DNA Repair** — Every day, your DNA takes hits from toxins, radiation, and metabolic stress. Normally, antioxidants and repair enzymes fix the damage. But nutrient deficiencies weaken these repair crews. Unrepaired DNA becomes mutations — the seed of cancer.
2. **Immune Surveillance** — The immune system is designed to spot and destroy abnormal cells. But stress, poor diet, and gut damage weaken immunity. Rogue cells escape detection.
3. **Growth Control** — Normal cells follow signals to stop dividing. Cancer cells ignore those signals. Animal proteins, IGF-1 (insulin-like growth factor), and inflammatory hormones tell them to keep growing.

Put simply: **cancer is normal biology gone unchecked because the terrain is compromised.**

The Terrain Connection

The modern diet creates perfect soil for tumors to grow:

- **Nutrient deficiencies** → weaken DNA repair, antioxidant defense, and immune cells.

- **Animal proteins** → overstimulate IGF-1, telling cancer cells to grow and divide.
- **Sugar overload** → feeds cancer cells directly; they thrive on glucose without normal metabolic brakes.
- **Toxins** → pesticides, preservatives, and chemicals damage DNA and overwhelm detox systems.
- **Inflammation** → chronic inflammation creates oxidative stress and fertile ground for tumor survival.

When the terrain is weak, cancer thrives. When the terrain is strong, cancer struggles.

The Antibiotic Connection

Most people don't realize antibiotics are linked to cancer growth. How?

1. **Microbiome Damage** — Antibiotics wipe out beneficial gut bacteria. Those bacteria regulate immunity, produce cancer-protective compounds like butyrate, and control inflammation. Without them, the immune system falters.
2. **Immune Suppression** — A disrupted microbiome weakens T-cells, the very soldiers that detect and kill rogue cells. Studies show repeated antibiotic use correlates with higher risk of colon, breast, and lung cancers.
3. **Direct Growth Effects** — Some studies stated antibiotics may alter mitochondrial function in ways that support tumor cell survival. The very drugs used casually for colds and infections may quietly cultivate the terrain for cancer.

Populations and Cancer

Cancer patterns prove lifestyle, not luck, drives disease.

- Western nations with diets heavy in meat, dairy, sugar, and processed food have the highest cancer rates in the world.
- Populations eating traditional diets rich in beans, grains, vegetables, and fruit show dramatically lower cancer rates.
- When those populations switch to Western diets, cancer rates soar within a generation.

If cancer were genetic, these shifts wouldn't happen so quickly. The difference isn't DNA. It's dinner.

Stories That Make It Real
Michael's Prostate Cancer

Michael was diagnosed with early-stage prostate cancer. His instinct was surgery. But he also shifted his lifestyle: no more dairy, no more red meat, no processed junk. He filled his meals with beans, greens, berries, and flax. Within a year, his PSA levels improved, his energy rose, and he regained confidence that he was fueling healing instead of fueling cancer.

Dana's Breast Cancer

Dana feared soy, believing the myth that it "causes breast cancer." But when she learned that soy's phytoestrogens bind to the beta receptor (regulated) instead of the alpha receptor (unregulated), she added tofu, tempeh, and edamame. Research showed soy lowered her recurrence risk. Her fear turned into empowerment — food was part of her recovery.

Cancer stories like these remind us: the terrain is not fixed. Change the terrain, and you change the outcome.

Antibiotics, Pharmaceuticals, and Cancer

Antibiotics are only one piece of the terrain puzzle. The broader pharmaceutical approach often worsens the very conditions it tries to manage.

- **Antibiotics** → destroy gut flora, weaken immune defenses, and leave DNA vulnerable.
- **Antacids and PPIs** → block stomach acid, impair nutrient absorption, and reduce protective compounds like magnesium and B12 — nutrients vital for DNA repair.
- **Statins** → deplete CoQ10, weakening mitochondria and slowing cellular energy defense.
- **Blood pressure drugs** → drain electrolytes and weaken vascular repair, creating hidden instability.

Instead of strengthening the terrain, pharmaceuticals often thin the foundation. A system already under stress is now more vulnerable to rogue cells taking root.

Plants as Cancer Medicine

The good news is powerful: plants don't just **prevent** cancer — they can help **reverse** its course. A plant-based diet changes the terrain in ways pharmaceuticals never can.

Cruciferous Vegetables

Broccoli, kale, cauliflower, cabbage, Brussels sprouts. These contain sulforaphane and indole-3-carbinol, which:

- Activate detox enzymes in the liver.
- Trigger cancer cells to self-destruct (apoptosis).
- Block angiogenesis (the growth of blood vessels that feed tumors).

Berries

Blueberries, raspberries, strawberries, blackberries. Rich in anthocyanins and ellagic acid, they:

- Neutralize free radicals before DNA is damaged.
- Inhibit cancer-promoting enzymes.
- Reduce estrogen-driven tumor growth.

Turmeric

Turmeric's active compound, curcumin, is one of the most studied natural cancer fighters. It:

- Reduces chronic inflammation (cancer's fertilizer).
- Blocks NF-kB, a master switch that turns on tumor-promoting genes.
- Enhances chemotherapy effectiveness while protecting normal cells.

Legumes

Beans, lentils, chickpeas, soy. Rich in fiber, isoflavones, and resistant starch, they:

- Bind toxins in the gut, reducing colon cancer risk.
- Balance estrogen activity by binding to the beta receptor (regulated, protective).
- Feed gut bacteria that produce butyrate, a compound that suppresses tumor growth.

Whole Grains and Seeds

Quinoa, oats, flax, chia. They:

- Provide lignans and phytosterols that reduce hormone-driven cancers.
- Offer soluble fiber that lowers cholesterol (reducing bile acid buildup linked to colon cancer).
- Deliver steady glucose release, starving cancer of sudden fuel spikes.

How Plants Reverse Cancer

Plants shift the body's terrain on every level:

- **Reduce Inflammation** → chronic inflammation is the spark that keeps tumors alive. Plants extinguish it.
- **Fuel Detox Pathways** → crucifers, garlic, and onions upregulate liver enzymes that clear carcinogens.
- **Repair DNA** → antioxidants from berries, grapes, and greens neutralize free radicals before mutations occur.
- **Balance Hormones** → soy, flax, and legumes modulate estrogen, lowering breast and prostate cancer risk.
- **Starve Tumors** → fiber stabilizes blood sugar, cutting cancer's favorite fuel source.
- **Rebuild Immunity** → micronutrients and phytonutrients strengthen natural killer cells that patrol for rogue cells.

No pill, drug, or operation works this comprehensively. Only whole plant foods supply this orchestra of defenses.

Stories That Make It Real
James's Colon Cancer Recovery

James, 59, was diagnosed with colon cancer after years of heavy meat and processed food consumption. Alongside medical treatment, he transitioned to a whole-food, plant-based diet: beans, lentils, cruciferous vegetables, and whole grains. Within months, his energy surged, inflammation markers dropped, and follow-up scans showed no new growth. His oncologist called it "remarkable." James called it "plants."

Marta's Breast Cancer Battle

Marta, 48, feared soy would worsen her breast cancer. But after reading research, she embraced tofu, tempeh, and edamame. These soy foods bound to the **beta receptor** instead of the alpha, regulating estrogen activity. Combined with cruciferous vegetables and flaxseed, Marta's terrain strengthened. Her recurrence risk lowered, her hot flashes eased, and her recovery improved.

Alan's Prostate Cancer Stabilization

Alan, 65, had rising PSA levels and a strong family history of prostate cancer. Doctors suggested aggressive monitoring and possible surgery. Instead, Alan shifted to a plant-based lifestyle rich in tomatoes, beans, and turmeric. His PSA stabilized, inflammation fell, and his doctor admitted the diet "likely slowed progression."

These stories aren't miracles. They are biology. When the terrain is changed, cancer cells lose their fuel.

Global Proof: Cancer and Diet

Across the world, the evidence is undeniable: diet dictates cancer risk.

- **Japan (before Westernization):** Traditional diets centered on rice, soy, vegetables, and fish resulted in low cancer rates. But as Western fast food spread, so did colon, breast, and prostate cancers. Within a generation, rates skyrocketed.
- **Rural China:** For decades, villagers ate mostly rice, vegetables, beans, and greens. Cancer was rare. When wealth introduced more meat, dairy, and processed oils, cancer became common.
- **Okinawa, Japan:** One of the world's longest-lived populations, the Okinawans thrived on purple sweet potatoes, bitter melon, soy, and vegetables. Their cancer rates were among the lowest globally — until diets shifted to meat and processed food.
- **Seventh-day Adventists (Loma Linda, California):** This plant-centered community has significantly lower cancer rates than the surrounding population. Vegans in this group have the lowest rates of all.

The pattern is clear: when plants dominate, cancer diminishes. When animal foods, sugar, and chemicals dominate, cancer explodes.

A Cancer-Prevention Food Plan

Here's how to strengthen terrain and reduce cancer risk every day:

Daily Foundations

- **Cruciferous Vegetables:** Aim for at least one serving daily. Broccoli, kale, cauliflower, Brussels sprouts.
- **Berries:** A cup of blueberries, raspberries, or strawberries supplies DNA-protective anthocyanins.
- **Legumes:** One cup of beans, lentils, or chickpeas supports hormone balance and gut health.
- **Whole Grains:** Brown rice, oats, quinoa, or barley provide fiber and slow glucose release.
- **Seeds:** Flax and chia for lignans, pumpkin and sunflower for minerals, sesame for calcium.

Weekly Boosters

- **Turmeric:** Add ½ teaspoon of turmeric with black pepper to meals several times a week.
- **Garlic and Onions:** Rich in sulfur compounds that detoxify carcinogens.
- **Tomatoes (cooked):** High in lycopene, protective against prostate and breast cancers.
- **Green Tea:** Catechins reduce oxidative stress and support immune surveillance, and can inhibit angiogenesis.

Lifestyle Keys

- **Avoid antibiotics.** Protect your microbiome as a frontline defense.
- **Eliminate dairy and animal proteins.** Prevent IGF-1 overdrive and hormone disruption.

- **Cut refined sugar.** Starve cancer cells of their favorite fuel.
- **Sweat daily.** Exercise reduces insulin resistance and strengthens immunity.
- **Sleep deeply.** The body repairs DNA and restores immune strength during rest.

More Stories That Make It Real
Karen's Ovarian Cancer Recovery Support

Karen, 52, underwent treatment for ovarian cancer. Alongside conventional therapy, she transitioned to a fully plant-based diet — crucifers, soy, turmeric, berries, and beans. Her oncologist noted her energy remained unusually high during chemotherapy, her recovery was faster, and her follow-up scans showed no recurrence. Karen believes food gave her the resilience medicine could not.

Daniel's Lung Cancer Terrain Shift

Daniel, 61, a former smoker, was diagnosed with early-stage lung cancer. Determined to fight, he quit processed food, embraced juicing greens, and ate beans, sweet potatoes, and whole grains daily. His doctors were surprised when his cancer stabilized. Daniel wasn't. He said: ***"I stopped feeding cancer and started feeding my body."***

Priya's Family Legacy

Priya lost both parents to colon cancer. Genetics terrified her. But she took a different path — daily beans, turmeric, leafy greens, and zero dairy. Now in her 40s, her screenings show no signs of cancer. She reframed her family legacy: genes load the gun, but lifestyle chooses whether it fires.

Expanded Key Takeaways

- **Cancer is not random.** It is the predictable outcome of weak terrain.
- **Antibiotics can fuel cancer** by destroying the microbiome and suppressing immunity.
- **Pharmaceuticals often weaken terrain** instead of strengthening it.
- **Plant-based diets prevent, slow, and sometimes reverse cancer.** Crucifers, berries, legumes, turmeric, flax, and whole grains are central.
- **Global populations prove it.** When plants dominate, cancer rates plummet.
- **Lifestyle is the trigger.** Choose not to pull it.

Action Steps

1. Add at least one cruciferous vegetable and one cup of berries daily.
2. Replace meat or dairy with beans, lentils, or tofu three times per week.
3. Sprinkle ground flaxseed or chia seeds on breakfast daily.
4. Use turmeric and garlic as regular seasonings.
5. Avoid unnecessary antibiotics and processed foods with chemical additives.

Closing Message

Cancer is not fate. It is not random bad luck. It is the body's alarm — ignored for too long, finally screaming.

The truth is simple: cancer grows in weak terrain. Antibiotics, toxins, animal protein, sugar, and pills weaken that terrain. Plants restore it.

In **Taste Versus Cancer**, I detailed how plant compounds block tumor growth and protect DNA. In **The P53 Diet & Lifestyle,** I showed how a plant-based life doesn't just prevent cancer — it can help reverse it.

This book simplifies the message: **cancer is not random. It is a lifestyle disease. And the lifestyle that prevents it is within your reach, on your plate, every day.**

Chapter 15

Eating Habits: Patterns That Heal or Harm

Most people think health is about individual meals. A salad one day, a pizza the next. But the truth is this: **your body doesn't measure you by single meals. It measures you by patterns.**

What you do daily becomes your terrain. A plant-centered salad once a week won't erase six days of fast food. A soda every day becomes a habit that rewires metabolism. Over years, these patterns decide whether you thrive or decline.

That's why habits matter more than diets. Diets are temporary. Habits are permanent. Diets end. Habits last.

If your habits build health, your body thanks you with energy, resilience, and longevity. If your habits build disease, your body protests with symptoms, ailments, and eventually, chronic illness.

The Tragedy of Eating Bad — Even With Cancer

In my book **Taste Versus Cancer,** I highlighted a heartbreaking reality: even after a cancer diagnosis, many people keep eating poorly. You might think a life-threatening disease would flip the switch instantly. But habits are powerful.

- Patients finish chemotherapy and go straight to fast food.
- Families bring fried chicken or processed casseroles to "comfort" cancer patients.
- Hospitals serve bacon, pudding cups, and Jell-O to people recovering from tumor surgeries.

It's not because people want to harm themselves. It's because habits override urgency. Culture, cravings, and patterns run deeper than fear.

The tragedy is this: people fight cancer with surgery and pills while still feeding it with meat, dairy, sugar, and processed oils. Instead of rebuilding the terrain, they keep fueling the fire.

Healing requires more than medicine. It requires new habits.

Harmful Eating Habits
Let's break down the most destructive patterns that quietly build disease:

1. Mindless Eating
Eating while scrolling, driving, or working means food goes down without awareness. The brain doesn't register fullness. The result? Overeating and poor digestion.

2. Late-Night Eating
Digestion slows at night. Eating heavy meals before bed spikes blood sugar, disrupts sleep, and stores calories as fat. The terrain is left inflamed and unhealed.

3. Fast Food Habits
Fast food isn't just "occasional treats." For many, it's daily ritual. Salt, oil, sugar, and chemicals overwhelm the body. Over time, arteries clog, inflammation rises, and cancer terrain builds.

4. Skipping Plants

When meat, dairy, and refined carbs dominate, vegetables, beans, and fruit vanish from the plate. Without fiber, antioxidants, and phytochemicals, the terrain loses its natural defense.

5. Sugar Drinks

Soda, energy drinks, "fruit juice" cocktails — they flood the system with empty calories, spiking insulin and fueling cancer cells directly. One soda a day doesn't feel like much, but in a year that's 30 pounds of pure sugar hitting the bloodstream.

These habits are rarely one-time mistakes. They're repeated patterns that silently erode the body until disease feels "sudden." But it was never sudden. It was cumulative.

Healing Eating Habits

The good news is simple: just as harmful habits create disease, healing habits create health.

1. Plant-Centered Plates

Make fruits, vegetables, legumes, nuts, and seeds the center of every plate. Meat, dairy, and processed foods should not "push plants aside." Plants must dominate the table.

2. Regular Meals

Skipping meals leads to blood sugar crashes and desperate cravings. Eating balanced plant-based meals at regular times provides steady energy.

3. Hydration First

Drinking water before meals reduces overeating and supports digestion. Often what we mistake for hunger is thirst.

4. Slow Eating

Chewing fully signals fullness to the brain and extracts nutrients more efficiently. Slow eating also makes food a mindful ritual instead of a rushed necessity.

5. Food Awareness

A simple question before every meal: ***Will this food heal me or harm me?*** That pause changes everything.

Culture, Family, and the Weight of Habit

Most eating isn't driven by hunger. It's driven by culture.

- **Celebrations** → cake at birthdays, meat at holidays, alcohol at parties.
- **Tradition** → "comfort foods" passed down through generations, often heavy in dairy, oil, and meat.
- **Stress and Boredom** → eating as distraction, not nourishment.
- **Family Influence** → people often eat what their family eats, even if it harms them, because rejecting food feels like rejecting love.

This is why change is hard, even when health is on the line. Food is more than calories — it's identity, memory, and belonging. To change eating habits, you must be willing to challenge culture.

Why People Don't Change — Even When Sick

In ***Taste Versus Cancer***, I described a sad but common reality: even patients with advanced cancer keep eating poorly. Why?

1. **Denial.** People tell themselves, "One meal won't matter." But one meal becomes habit, and habit shapes terrain.
2. **Comfort.** Illness is frightening. People cling to familiar foods for emotional relief, even if those foods worsen their disease.

3. **Confusion.** Marketing convinces people yogurt is healthy, meat builds strength, or "low fat" snacks are healing. They don't realize they're feeding the illness.
4. **Inertia.** Habits have momentum. It feels easier to keep doing what you've always done than to change.
5. **Environment.** Hospitals, family gatherings, and workplaces still serve processed, animal-heavy food — reinforcing destructive patterns.

The result is tragic: people literally feed cancer while trying to fight it. Pills and surgeries may treat tumors, but daily food fuels either recovery or relapse.

Stories That Make It Real
Clara's Recovery from Comfort Eating

Clara, 58, battled breast cancer. After each treatment session, family and friends brought casseroles filled with cheese and cream to "cheer her up." She kept eating them, thinking food was comfort. But her weight rose, her energy dropped, and her digestion worsened. When she shifted to plant-based soups, greens, and beans, her recovery improved and her energy soared. She realized comfort food should **comfort health, not destroy it.**

Eddie's Late-Night Habit

Eddie, 45, was diagnosed with colon cancer. Even after surgery, he snacked on processed meat sandwiches late at night, convinced it was harmless. His digestive pain worsened. A plant-based coach taught him to replace late meals with calming herbal teas and fruit earlier in the evening. Within weeks, his symptoms improved and his sleep deepened.

Nina's Sugar Cravings

Nina, 37, couldn't stop drinking soda, even during chemotherapy. She admitted it was the only thing that "gave her joy." Her doctor begged her to quit. Only after she joined a plant-based support group did she find healthier swaps — sparkling water with lemon and fresh fruit smoothies. Her cravings dropped, and so did her treatment side effects.

These stories show the pull of habit. Even in crisis, food choices remain tethered to culture, comfort, and craving. But they also prove change is possible — when awareness grows.

Practical Strategies to Replace Harmful Habits

Breaking harmful patterns isn't about willpower. It's about replacement.

- **Mindless Snacking → Mindful Eating.** Instead of chips at the TV, keep cut fruit or veggie sticks ready. Eat without screens.
- **Late-Night Eating → Soothing Rituals.** Replace food with calming tea, stretching, or journaling before bed.
- **Fast Food → Fast Plants.** Prepare beans, lentils, and chopped veggies in bulk. Make "grab-and-go" meals plant-based.
- **Sugar Drinks → Natural Hydration.** Carry a reusable bottle. Flavor water with berries, lemon, or mint.
- **Skipping Plants → Anchoring with Greens.** Commit to one salad, one fruit, and one bean dish every day, no matter what else happens.

Habits don't vanish by force. They're swapped. Healing begins when you trade a disease-feeding habit for a health-feeding one.

A Step-by-Step Plan for Habit Transformation

Changing eating habits can feel overwhelming, but the process becomes simple when broken into steps.

Step 1: Identify Your Most Harmful Habit

Is it soda? Fast food? Late-night eating? Skipping vegetables? Pick one. Not all. One.

Step 2: Ask the Healing Question

Before each meal, pause and ask: ***Will this food heal me or harm me?*** That moment of awareness interrupts autopilot eating.

Step 3: Replace, Don't Remove

Swap soda for sparkling water, chips for almonds, fast food for a bean-and-veggie wrap. Removing without replacing leads to relapse.

Step 4: Anchor New Habits with Routines

- Start the day with fruit.
- Add greens to lunch.
- Make beans or lentils part of dinner.
  Anchors create momentum.

Step 5: Build Support

Habits are reinforced by environment. Join a plant-based group. Share meals with friends who support change. Stock your home with real food.

Step 6: Celebrate Progress, Not Perfection

One bad meal doesn't undo the pattern. Health is cumulative. Each healing choice is a deposit into your future.

Expanded Key Takeaways

- **Health is not built by one meal — it's built by habits.**
- **Harmful habits** include late-night eating, fast food, sugar drinks, and skipping plants.
- **Healing habits** include plant-centered plates, mindful eating, hydration, and routine.
- **Culture drives habits,** but you can rewrite culture by choosing different foods daily.
- **Even cancer patients often keep harmful habits,** but those who shift to plant-based healing regain energy and resilience.
- **Habits can be replaced.** Awareness plus substitution builds long-term change.

Action Steps

1. Write down your top three harmful eating habits. Circle the one you'll change first.
2. Create one swap today: soda → water, fast food → beans, chips → fruit.
3. Start a food journal for one week. Note not just what you eat, but when, where, and why. Patterns will emerge.
4. Build one anchor habit this week: fruit at breakfast, salad at lunch, beans at dinner.

Closing Message

Your health is not a single event. It is a pattern.

In **Taste Versus Cancer**, I showed how heartbreaking it is that people continue to eat poorly even after cancer strikes — proving that habits, not fear, drive choices. In **The P53 Diet & Lifestyle,** I explained how daily patterns shape terrain more than isolated meals.

This book simplifies the truth: **habits build terrain. Terrain builds health.**

The good news is, you hold the pen. Each meal is a line. Each day is a paragraph. Over time, your habits write the story of your health.

The question is simple: will your habits tell a story of healing — or harm?

Chapter 16

Problems with Pills & Supplements

We live in a **pill bottle culture.** Every problem has a capsule.

- Headache? Take a pain pill.
- Heartburn? Swallow an antacid.
- Fatigue? Pop caffeine pills.
- High cholesterol? Grab a statin.
- High blood pressure? Take a diuretic.
- Nutrient gaps? Swallow a multivitamin.

Relief is instant. But relief is not healing. Pills do not create health — they mask symptoms, silence alarms, and postpone the real work of root-cause healing.

Supplements join the illusion. Advertisements promise "insurance" in a bottle: one capsule to cover all your nutritional sins. But the truth is, isolated powders and extracts can never replace the synergy of real food.

The truth is simple: **pills manage disease, but they don't build wellness.**

The Problem with Pills

Prescription drugs can help in emergencies. But as a lifestyle, they fail.

1. **Masking Symptoms**

   Pills silence signals without solving causes. A painkiller quiets the headache but doesn't fix dehydration. An antacid calms heartburn but hides the inflammation caused by dairy and oils.

2. **Side Effects and New Pills**

   Every pill carries side effects, and those side effects often require more pills. A blood pressure drug causes fatigue → a stimulant is prescribed. A painkiller damages the stomach → an antacid is added. Soon patients take five, ten, even fifteen pills daily.

3. **Nutrient Depletion**

   Many common drugs strip nutrients from the body — leaving terrain weaker over time.

   - Diuretics → drain magnesium, potassium, and zinc.
   - Statins → deplete CoQ10, critical for energy.
   - Antacids → block absorption of iron, calcium, and B12.
   - Antibiotics → wipe out gut flora that produce vitamins.

Instead of healing, pills create hidden deficiencies that worsen disease.

1. **Dependency**

   Pills encourage dependency. Instead of changing diet or lifestyle, patients rely on daily refills. The body adapts, side effects build, and the root cause grows deeper.

Pills manage illness. They rarely build wellness.

The Problem with Supplements

Supplements are marketed as the safe alternative to drugs. But they carry their own problems.

1. **Poor Absorption**
   Most supplements are not absorbed the way natural food is. Calcium carbonate, for example, often passes through the gut unabsorbed. Iron supplements cause constipation without improving status if the body lacks cofactors.

2. **Contamination**
   Many supplements, especially cheap brands, are con- taminated with heavy metals, pesticides, or fillers. Independent tests regularly expose protein powders laced with lead, or herbal capsules spiked with unde- clared pharmaceuticals.

3. **Isolated Nutrients**
   Supplements deliver single chemicals, divorced from the web of co-factors that make nutrients work in na- ture. A vitamin C pill lacks the flavonoids in an or- ange that enhance absorption. An iron pill lacks the copper and vitamin C needed to use it properly.

4. **False Confidence**
   Perhaps the greatest danger is psychological. People eat poorly, assuming supplements are "insurance." They believe a pill covers their processed food, sugar, and meat — but no capsule can undo that damage.

5. **Overdoses and Imbalances**

- Fat-soluble vitamins (A, D, E, K) accumulate and cause toxicity.
- High-dose antioxidants can actually promote cancer by disrupting natural cell signaling.
- Imbalanced formulas deplete other nutrients (for example, too much zinc suppresses copper).

In my research on supplements, I detailed case after case of how they disappoint or even harm.

The Food Advantage

Food is not just nutrients. Food is synergy.

- A blueberry isn't just vitamin C. It's C plus anthocyanins, polyphenols, fiber, water, and hundreds of phytochemicals working together.
- A walnut isn't just omega-3 fat. It's minerals, antioxidants, protein, and fiber in perfect natural proportion.
- A lentil isn't just protein. It's iron, folate, magnesium, and resistant starch that feed gut bacteria.

No supplement can replicate this orchestra. Pills are single notes. Plants are symphonies.

Stories That Make It Real
Mark's Multivitamin Myth

Mark, 42, ate fast food daily but took a multivitamin "for balance." He believed the pill protected him. At 50, he had a heart attack. Doctors explained vitamins can't cancel burgers. He now thrives on beans, greens, and fruit — no multivitamin required.

Sophie's Energy Supplements

Sophie, 34, spent hundreds on "energy" supplements — ginseng, B12 shots, caffeine pills. Yet fatigue persisted. When she switched to a plant-based diet with beans, greens, fruit, and nuts, her energy soared. No pill matched the power of food.

Henry's Statin Struggles

Henry, 60, took statins for cholesterol. His LDL dropped, but he developed muscle pain and fatigue. He later learned statins depleted his CoQ10. When he transitioned to oats, beans, nuts, and vegetables, his cholesterol normalized without side effects.

Alicia's Antacids

Alicia lived on antacids for reflux. She thought she had a "pill deficiency." In reality, dairy and fried food caused the problem. When she removed them and ate greens, beans, and whole grains, her reflux disappeared — and so did her dependency.

The Cycle of Pharma Dependency vs. Food Empowerment

Pills create a **trap.** A symptom appears, a pill is prescribed. The symptom quiets, but the cause grows. Side effects show up. Another pill is prescribed. Soon, one problem becomes five — not because the body is failing, but because the root cause was never addressed.

- **High blood pressure** → diuretic → nutrient loss → cramps → muscle relaxer → fatigue → stimulant.
- **High cholesterol** → statin → CoQ10 depletion → fatigue and muscle pain → painkillers.
- **Reflux** → antacid → nutrient depletion → anemia → iron pill → constipation.

This domino effect is not rare — it is standard. Millions of people become dependent on a web of pills that weaken them more over time.

Food breaks the cycle. A plant-based diet nourishes terrain, removes causes, and strengthens systems. Instead of stacking pills, you build resilience.

The Most Abused Supplements

Not all supplements are harmful in all cases, but many are abused, misunderstood, or marketed with false promises.

1. Multivitamins

Marketed as "insurance," but they give false confidence. They often contain synthetic forms (like folic acid instead of natural folate) that are poorly used by the body. Studies show little benefit for chronic disease prevention.

2. Protein Powders

The obsession with protein has made powders a billion-dollar business. Yet most people already get enough protein — often too much. Powders often:

- Contain heavy metal contamination (lead, arsenic, cadmium).
- Deliver isolated amino acids that spike IGF-1, fueling cancer growth.
- Replace real food with artificial shakes.

3. Fish Oil

Once hailed as a heart-protective miracle, research now shows mixed or even harmful results. Fish oil oxidizes easily, creating free radicals. Meanwhile, fish themselves accumulate mercury, PCBs, and microplastics. Whole plant sources (flax, chia, hemp, walnuts) provide omega-3s safely.

4. Vitamin D Megadoses

Vitamin D deficiency is real, especially in low-sun regions. But high-dose supplements can cause calcium imbalances, kidney stones, and vascular calcification. The better long-term solution is modest supplementation if needed, combined with sunlight and plant-based diet support.

5. "Energy Boosters"

Caffeine pills, "B-complex shots," and stimulant blends don't provide energy — they borrow it. The crash always comes. Real energy comes from mitochondrial health, fueled by whole plants, not stimulants.

Why Supplements Can't Replace Food

Supplements isolate. Food integrates.

- A pill of vitamin C provides one molecule. An orange provides vitamin C plus hesperidin, rutin, naringenin, fiber, water, and dozens of synergistic compounds.
- A calcium tablet may not absorb. Kale provides calcium plus vitamin K, magnesium, and phytonutrients that guide it to bones.
- A protein shake is stripped and denatured. Lentils offer protein alongside iron, folate, fiber, and resistant starch.

The human body evolved with whole food. Supplements are fragments pretending to be complete.

More Stories That Make It Real
Tom's Protein Powder Addiction

Tom, 28, lived at the gym and drank three protein shakes daily.

He felt strong, but bloodwork revealed high LDL and early kidney strain. When he swapped powders for beans, quinoa, and nuts, his strength remained — but his labs improved dramatically.

Maria's Multivitamin Illusion

Maria, 50, believed her daily multivitamin protected her while she ate processed food. She was shocked when diagnosed with prediabetes and high blood pressure. A health coach helped her transition to plant-based meals. Within a year, she reversed both conditions. The vitamin had done nothing. Plants did everything.

George and the Fish Oil Fiasco

George, 65, took fish oil capsules for years. Yet his heart disease progressed. He later learned fish oil oxidizes easily, especially in cheap capsules. When he switched to walnuts, flax, and chia, his triglycerides dropped and inflammation markers improved.

Helen's Antacid Dependency

Helen, 47, lived on antacids for reflux. Her doctor added calcium supplements after bone scans showed weakening. What she didn't know: her antacids blocked calcium absorption in the first place. Once she cut dairy and oils and ate greens and beans, her reflux disappeared — and her bone density improved without pills.

Food as Empowerment

The most powerful shift isn't just physical. It's psychological.

- Pills create dependence: you wait for a doctor, a refill, an external fix.

- Food creates empowerment: you control what enters your mouth, your cells, your terrain.

This is why people who shift to whole-food, plant-based eating often describe more than improved labs. They describe freedom.

A Step-by-Step Guide to Moving Away from Pill Dependency

Changing from a pill-based life to a plant-based one doesn't happen overnight. But step by step, you can move from dependency to empowerment.

Step 1: Audit Your Pills and Supplements

Write down every prescription drug, over-the-counter pill, and supplement you take. Ask yourself:

- Why am I taking this?
- Does it solve the cause or just mask the symptom?
- What nutrients might this deplete?

Step 2: Ask Your Provider the Right Questions

Bring the list to your doctor and ask:

- "Do I still need this?"
- "What lifestyle changes could reduce my need for this pill?"
- "What nutrient deficiencies could this drug cause?"

Step 3: Replace, Don't Just Remove

Don't quit cold turkey without support. Instead:

- Replace antacids with a plant-based diet that removes reflux triggers.

- Replace cholesterol drugs with beans, oats, nuts, and seeds that lower LDL naturally.
- Replace energy supplements with whole-food carbohydrates, hydration, and rest.

Step 4: Build Anchors in Food

- Fruit for breakfast.
- Beans or lentils at lunch.
- Greens at dinner.
  These anchors stabilize blood sugar, energy, and digestion — the very areas pills usually target.

Step 5: Track Improvements

Keep a journal of symptoms, energy, digestion, and sleep. Most people notice improvements within weeks of replacing pills with plants.

Step 6: Trust the Process

Health doesn't come from bottles. It comes from patterns. Be patient, consistent, and aware.

Expanded Key Takeaways

- **Pills manage symptoms but rarely heal causes.** They often create side effects and nutrient depletion.
- **Supplements are not insurance.** They are often poorly absorbed, contaminated, or misleading.
- **Food provides synergy.** No pill replicates the orchestra of compounds in plants.
- **The cycle of dependency can be broken.** Replace pills with food, not just willpower.
- **Empowerment begins at the plate.** You are not at the mercy of pills; you are in charge of your terrain.

Action Steps

1. Audit your pills and supplements today.
2. Replace one supplement with a whole-food source this week (flax instead of fish oil, kale instead of calcium tablets).
3. Add one food anchor daily: fruit, beans, or greens.
4. Start a "pill reduction journal" with your provider's guidance.
5. Consult with your doctor first.

Closing Message

Pills manage disease. Plants create health.

Supplements may fill narrow gaps, but they cannot replace the synergy of whole food. Pills may save lives in emergencies, but they are not the foundation of wellness.

In my research on pharmaceuticals, in my book ***How You Are Being Poisoned,*** I showed how common drugs deplete nutrients and create new deficiencies. **In *The P53 Diet & Lifestyle,*** I explained how real healing happens when we nourish the terrain with plants.

This book keeps the message clear: **health is not in a pill bottle. Health is on your plate.**

Chapter 17

Exercise: Movement as Medicine

Picture your ancestors. They didn't sit at desks for eight hours, then drive home to collapse on a couch. They walked, climbed, carried, hunted, and gathered. Movement wasn't optional — it was survival.

Today, the opposite is true. Cars replace walking. Machines replace lifting. Screens replace play. Our bodies were built for motion, yet we live in stillness.

And stillness is killing us.

The World Health Organization calls inactivity one of the leading causes of chronic disease worldwide. Sitting is now compared to smoking in terms of health risk. Lack of movement leads to heart disease, diabetes, cancer, depression, and premature death.

The truth is simple: **exercise is medicine.** Not in a pill. Not in a bottle. But in the daily rhythm of movement.

Why Movement Heals

Exercise isn't just about burning calories. It transforms your body at every level:

- **Heart and Circulation** – Strengthens the heart, lowers blood pressure, improves blood flow.
- **Metabolism** – Increases insulin sensitivity, stabilizes blood sugar, reduces diabetes risk.
- **Immune System** – Enhances surveillance, helping your body spot and destroy rogue cells (including cancer).
- **Hormones** – Balances cortisol (stress), boosts serotonin and dopamine (mood), increases growth hormone (repair).
- **Brain** – Stimulates new brain cells, improves memory, lowers risk of dementia.
- **Longevity** – Every hour of moderate exercise adds hours back to your life.

No pill, supplement, or treatment offers these benefits all at once. Only movement does.

The Neutral Effect Without Plants

Here's what most people miss: **exercise alone isn't enough.**

If you exercise daily but fuel with meat, dairy, processed oils, and sugar, your gains are neutralized. You may build muscle, but you're also building plaque. You may strengthen lungs, but you're feeding inflammation. You may sweat out stress, but you're still fueling cancer cells with animal protein and refined glucose.

Think of it this way: exercise is the spark. Food is the fuel. If the fuel is toxic, the spark does little. If the fuel is pure, the spark ignites healing.

This is why so many athletes — runners, weightlifters, even weekend warriors — still suffer from heart attacks, diabetes, and cancer. Exercise cannot override a toxic diet. At best, it delays the consequences. At worst, it masks them until it's too late.

In *The P53 Diet & Lifestyle,* I stressed this truth: **movement has power only when paired with plants.** Together, they build terrain that resists disease.

The Mental Health Connection

Exercise is one of the most powerful antidepressants known.

A brisk 30-minute walk can reduce anxiety as effectively as medication — without side effects. Regular activity boosts serotonin, dopamine, and endorphins, rewiring the brain toward calm and joy.

But again, diet matters. Exercise plus processed food may lift mood temporarily, but blood sugar crashes drag you down. Exercise plus plants stabilizes the brain with steady fuel and nutrients.

Movement is not just physical medicine. It's emotional and mental medicine too.

The Myth of Intensity

Many people avoid exercise because they think it has to be extreme: marathons, CrossFit, bootcamps. But the truth is, movement doesn't need to be complicated or punishing.

Walking, gardening, dancing, yoga, swimming — all count. The key is consistency, not intensity.

And here's another myth: "I can exercise hard to earn junk food." The truth is, you cannot out-train a bad diet. Junk food cancels gains. Plant food amplifies them.

In *The P53 Diet & Lifestyle,* I explained that 30–60 minutes of moderate activity most days is enough to transform health. You don't need an expensive gym membership. You just need to move — and to fuel that movement with plants.

Movement Without Plants vs. Movement With Plants

People often assume exercise alone guarantees health. But here's the truth: **exercise in the wrong terrain produces limited or even neutral effects.**

- A runner who fuels with bacon and eggs may have strong legs but clogged arteries.
- A gym-goer who chugs protein shakes may build muscle but also feed cancer growth with excess IGF-1.
- A cyclist who downs energy gels and sodas may pedal for hours but still fuel diabetes with sugar spikes.

The terrain matters more than the movement. **You cannot out-train a toxic diet.**

By contrast, when movement is paired with a plant-based diet:

- Blood vessels stay flexible and clean.
- The immune system is stronger, spotting and destroying rogue cells.
- Inflammation is lowered, making recovery faster and joints more resilient.
- Cancer-fueling pathways (IGF-1, oxidative stress, DNA damage) are downregulated.
- Exercise feels easier because the body runs on clean fuel.

This is why plant-based athletes — from ultra-marathoners to strength trainers — consistently show faster recovery, reduced inflammation, and longer careers.

Movement and Disease Prevention

Exercise has proven benefits, but its full power shines only when diet supports it.

- **Heart Disease** → Regular exercise lowers risk by 35–40%. But in meat-eaters, plaques still form. In plant-based eaters, exercise plus plants not only prevents but can reverse arterial damage.
- **Type 2 Diabetes** → Exercise improves insulin sensitivity immediately, even after one session. But if paired with processed junk, the benefit fades. With whole-food carbs, insulin sensitivity compounds.
- **Cancer** → Active people have lower risk, but cancer still thrives in toxic terrain. Only when exercise is paired with crucifers, berries, legumes, and fiber does the terrain shift strongly against tumors.
- **Dementia** → Exercise boosts blood flow to the brain. Plants add antioxidants that protect neurons. Together, they provide the sharpest shield.
- **Depression** → Exercise lifts mood. Plants stabilize it with steady glucose and serotonin precursors like tryptophan.

Movement is a prescription. Plants are the delivery system. Without both, healing is incomplete.

Stories That Make It Real
Brian's Marathon Wake-Up Call

Brian, 44, was a marathon runner. Friends called him the picture of health. But one morning, after training, he collapsed with chest pain. Doctors found arterial blockages. His running couldn't undo years of steak, eggs, and butter. When Brian adopted a plant-based diet, his arteries began to heal. Running became healing instead of harm.

Laura's Fitness Plateau

Laura, 36, loved yoga and spin classes. Yet she constantly battled fatigue and struggled with weight. She drank protein shakes daily, convinced they were necessary. When she switched to lentils, beans, and greens, her energy soared, her weight dropped, and her yoga practice deepened. Exercise plus plants unlocked her potential.

Sam's Cancer Recovery Support

Sam, 59, had prostate cancer. He walked daily, hoping it would help. It did — but only modestly. His doctor told him movement was good, but diet mattered more. When Sam gave up meat and embraced beans, crucifers, and berries, his energy improved and his PSA stabilized. Movement without plants had been neutral. Movement with plants became transformative.

Practical "Movement + Food" Combinations

- **Pre-exercise fuel:** Bananas, dates, or oatmeal provide steady glucose without spikes.
- **Post-exercise recovery:** Smoothie with berries, spinach, flaxseed, and plant milk supplies antioxidants, protein, and anti-inflammatory compounds.
- **Daily base fuel:** Beans, whole grains, and greens stabilize blood sugar and provide glycogen stores for endurance.
- **Joint protection:** Cruciferous vegetables and turmeric reduce inflammation, making workouts easier and safer.

Think of it this way: **exercise primes the body. Plants provide the materials.** Without both, the house never gets built.

A Step-by-Step Plan for Plant-Powered Movement

Step 1: Anchor Plants First

Movement draws energy from whatever you fuel it with. Begin by anchoring every day with plant-based meals:

- Fruit for breakfast.
- Beans or lentils at lunch.
- Greens at dinner.

Step 2: Choose Joyful Movement

The best exercise is the one you'll actually do. Walking, dancing, gardening, cycling, yoga — all count. Consistency matters more than intensity.

Step 3: Pair Food with Movement

- Pre-workout: bananas, dates, or oatmeal for steady glucose.
- Post-workout: berries, spinach, flax, and plant protein from legumes or nuts.
  This pairing repairs muscles, replenishes glycogen, and fights inflammation.

Step 4: Mix Strength, Cardio, and Flexibility

- Strength → bodyweight, resistance bands, or weights 2–3x weekly.
- Cardio → brisk walking, swimming, cycling.

· Flexibility → yoga, tai chi, or stretching.
Plants fuel all three without baggage from cholesterol or saturated fat.

Step 5: Track How You Feel

Notice changes in energy, sleep, mood, and recovery. Plant-powered movement often produces faster improvements than exercise alone.

Step 6: Let Movement and Plants Reinforce Each Other

The more you move, the more plants you'll crave. The more plants you eat, the more you'll want to move. This cycle builds resilience.

Expanded Key Takeaways

- **Your body was built to move.** Stillness breeds disease, movement breeds life.
- **Exercise is medicine — but not in isolation.** Without plants, exercise has a neutral or even negative effect.
- **Movement transforms every system:** heart, brain, hormones, immunity, metabolism.
- **You cannot out-train a toxic diet.** Exercise plus meat, dairy, and junk food leaves terrain vulnerable.
- **Plant-based fuel amplifies exercise benefits.** It lowers inflammation, strengthens immunity, and protects DNA.
- **Consistency matters more than intensity.** Daily movement, even moderate, builds lasting health.

Action Steps

1. Walk 30 minutes today — outside if possible.
2. Replace pre-workout processed snacks with bananas, oats, or dates.
3. Drink a smoothie with greens and berries after exercise.
4. Try one strength activity this week — push-ups, squats, or resistance bands.
5. Track energy and mood for 7 days of plant-powered movement.

Closing Message

You don't need a prescription for health. You need permission to move — and to fuel that movement with plants.

The truth is simple: **exercise is medicine, but only when fueled by the right diet.** Movement alone can delay disease, but paired with a plant-based lifestyle, it reverses it.

In ***The P53 Diet & Lifestyle,*** I explained how exercise enhances immunity, metabolism, and mental health — but only in synergy with plant foods. In ***Understanding Hormones, Enzymes, and Cell Receptors***, I showed how movement regulates cortisol, insulin, and growth hormone — but again, food determines the terrain.

This book keeps the message clear: **exercise is not optional, and neither is diet. Movement is the spark. Plants are the fuel. Together, they create healing.**

Chapter 18

Herbs & Spices: Nature's Hidden Healers

Herbs and spices don't take up much space on your plate. A sprinkle here, a pinch there. No bulk like grains, no fiber like beans, no calories to fill you up. And yet, they are among the most concentrated healing agents in the plant kingdom.

For centuries, cultures used herbs and spices as medicine before pills ever existed. Turmeric for inflammation, garlic for immunity, cinnamon for blood sugar, oregano for infections. Today, modern science is catching up — proving that the smallest flavors often deliver the biggest healing power.

Small but mighty, herbs and spices pack phytochemicals, antioxidants, and compounds that transform ordinary meals into medicine.

Why Herbs and Spices Heal

Herbs and spices deliver what many other foods cannot: **ultra-concentrated plant chemistry.**

- **Antioxidants:** Polyphenols, carotenoids, and flavonoids that quench free radicals before they damage DNA.
- **Anti-inflammatory compounds:** Curcumin (turmeric), allicin (garlic), capsaicin (chili peppers).
- **Immune regulators:** Garlic, oregano, and ginger stimulate immune cells while calming harmful over-reactions.
- **Blood sugar control:** Cinnamon and fenugreek improve insulin sensitivity.
- **Circulatory protection:** Garlic, turmeric, and cayenne improve blood flow and prevent clotting.

Unlike synthetic drugs, herbs and spices deliver these compounds in synergy — working with the body instead of against it.

Keep Salt Down

One seasoning deserves caution: salt.

Sodium is essential in small amounts, but the modern diet overloads it. Processed food, fast food, and restaurant meals can easily push sodium intake to 3,000–5,000 mg per day — more than double or triple the safe amount.

Excess sodium contributes to:

- High blood pressure
- Kidney damage
- Fluid retention
- Stroke and heart disease

The solution is simple: **keep salt under 1,200 mg per day.**

Flavor your food with herbs and spices instead: garlic, basil, oregano, cumin, turmeric, rosemary, ginger, chili peppers, parsley, and cilantro. They transform food while protecting your arteries, heart, and brain.

Cancer-Fighting Herbs and Spices
Turmeric

- Contains curcumin, one of the most studied natural anti-cancer compounds.
- Reduces inflammation, blocks tumor blood supply (angiogenesis), and promotes apoptosis (self-destruction of abnormal cells).

Garlic & Onions

- Rich in allicin and sulfur compounds.
- Detoxify carcinogens, regulate estrogen metabolism, and improve immune surveillance.
- Populations that consume garlic regularly show lower rates of stomach and colon cancer.

Ginger

- Contains gingerol, which slows cancer cell proliferation.
- Reduces nausea and calms systemic inflammation, aiding both prevention and recovery.

Cinnamon

- Improves blood sugar control, reducing insulin spikes that feed cancer cells.

· Contains cinnamaldehyde, which blocks abnormal signaling in tumor cells.

Rosemary & Oregano

· Packed with rosmarinic acid and carnosol, both shown to slow tumor growth.
· Potent antibacterial and antiviral activity that supports immune strength.

Chili Peppers

· Capsaicin disrupts cancer cell metabolism and promotes apoptosis.
· Also stimulates metabolism, aiding weight management.

The Ailment Connection

Herbs and spices don't just defend against cancer — they ease everyday ailments, often where pills only mask symptoms:

· **Cinnamon** – Balances blood sugar, helping reverse Type 2 diabetes.
· **Ginger** – Calms nausea, arthritis pain, and gut inflammation.
· **Garlic** – Drops blood pressure naturally and supports cholesterol balance.
· **Peppermint** – Soothes IBS symptoms and aids digestion.
· **Turmeric** – Reduces joint pain, stiffness, and systemic inflammation.

Instead of silencing the body with pills, herbs and spices correct the imbalance.

Stories That Make It Real
Angela's Arthritis Relief

Angela, 64, suffered from aching joints for years. Pain pills upset her stomach, leaving her stuck between pain and side effects. When she began adding turmeric and black pepper to her meals daily, the pain subsided within weeks. Her morning stiffness decreased, and she regained mobility without needing another pill.

Sam's Blood Pressure Victory

Sam, 55, was told blood pressure pills would be lifelong. Instead, he cut processed food, slashed salt, and seasoned his meals with garlic, oregano, and cumin. Within three months, his blood pressure dropped naturally. His doctor reduced his medication, stunned by the results. Sam's story proves: flavor can replace pharmaceuticals.

Priya's Cancer Recovery Support

During breast cancer treatment, Priya added turmeric, ginger, and garlic daily alongside her plant-based diet. Her oncologist noted her resilience, faster healing, and reduced inflammatory markers. Priya says, *"The food was my daily medicine. It helped me feel like I had power in the fight."*

Diego's Diabetes Reversal

Diego, 49, had struggled with Type 2 diabetes for a decade. When he began sprinkling cinnamon into his oatmeal, drinking cinnamon tea, and using fenugreek seeds, his blood sugar stabilized. Combined with a P53 plant-based pattern, his A1C numbers improved, and he eventually came off insulin altogether.

How Herbs and Spices Work in the Body

It's not magic. It's chemistry — powerful plant chemistry interacting with human biology.

Turmeric (Curcumin)

· Suppresses NF-κB, a molecular switch that drives inflammation.
· Inhibits angiogenesis — the creation of blood vessels that feed tumors.
· Encourages apoptosis, the "suicide" program that clears damaged cells.

Garlic (Allicin & Sulfur Compounds)

· Boosts glutathione, the body's master antioxidant.
· Enhances liver detoxification pathways, removing carcinogens.
· Naturally thins the blood, reducing clot risk without side effects.

Cinnamon (Cinnamaldehyde & Polyphenols)

· Increases glucose uptake in muscle cells.
· Mimics insulin activity, improving sensitivity and lowering blood sugar.
· Blocks oxidative stress that damages pancreatic beta cells.

Ginger (Gingerol & Shogaol)

· Reduces prostaglandins, compounds that trigger pain and swelling.
· Calms nausea by interacting with serotonin receptors in the gut.
· Inhibits cancer cell signaling pathways.

Chili Peppers (Capsaicin)

· Activates TRPV1 receptors, releasing endorphins and lowering pain.
· Forces cancer cells into metabolic stress, leading to apoptosis.
· Boosts thermogenesis, increasing fat burning and energy balance.

These are not fringe claims — these are documented biochemical pathways, showing how the smallest herbs can trigger powerful healing.

Cultural Wisdom: Herbs in Longevity Traditions
India — Ayurveda

For thousands of years, turmeric, ginger, cumin, and fenugreek have been staples of Ayurvedic medicine. Today, we know these spices reduce inflammation, balance blood sugar, and protect DNA. Curry powders weren't just flavor — they were pharmacy.

Mediterranean — Herbs of the Blue Zone

Ikaria, Greece, is famous for its longevity. Daily, the Ikarians consume oregano, rosemary, sage, and garlic in teas, soups, and stews. These herbs deliver antioxidants, lower blood pressure, and improve circulation. Their kitchen gardens are medicine chests.

China — Traditional Chinese Medicine

Ginger, garlic, ginseng, and licorice root have been prescribed for centuries to balance energy, strengthen immunity, and regulate digestion. Modern research confirms their bioactive compounds protect against chronic disease.

Latin America — Spice and Heat

In Mexico and Central America, chili peppers, cumin, and cinnamon are daily staples. Capsaicin from chilies keeps blood flow-ing, fights infections, and revs metabolism. Cinnamon stabilizes sugar from staples like corn and beans.

Middle East – Healing Flavors

Coriander, cumin, garlic, and parsley dominate Middle Eastern cooking. These spices balance hormones, cleanse toxins, and protect heart health. Many of the world's oldest written recipes doubled as medical prescriptions.

Why Herbs & Spices Are Undervalued Today

So why don't we hear more about them? Because you can't patent turmeric. You can't trademark garlic. There's no profit in cinnamon tea or rosemary sprigs.

Instead, the food and pharmaceutical industries keep people hooked on pills and processed food while dismissing herbs as "alternative." But the truth is the opposite: **herbs and spices were the original medicine, and science continues to prove their value.**

Practical Ways to Use More Herbs & Spices

Herbs and spices don't work if they sit in the cupboard. Their power comes from daily use — small, consistent amounts layered into meals.

1. Swap Salt for Flavor

- Replace salt shakers with garlic powder, onion powder, smoked paprika, lemon, and herbs.
- Use spice blends instead of sodium-heavy sauces.
- Train your taste buds — within weeks, food tastes vibrant without excess salt.

2. Spice Breakfast

- Add cinnamon to oats, smoothies, or fruit for blood sugar control.
- Ginger tea or turmeric lattes are morning medicine in a cup.
- Fresh mint in water wakes up digestion.

3. Cook with Turmeric

- Stir into soups, stews, curries, or roasted vegetables.
- Always add black pepper — it boosts curcumin absorption by 2,000%.

4. Fresh Herbs Daily

- Keep parsley, cilantro, basil, or dill in your kitchen.
- Chop and sprinkle on meals — raw herbs preserve antioxidants lost in cooking.

5. Tea Time

- Herbal teas double as medicine: ginger for digestion, peppermint for calm, cinnamon for balance, hibiscus for blood pressure.
- Green tea has been shown to inhibit angiogenesis.

6. Go Global for Inspiration

- Learn from cultural traditions:
  - Indian curries with turmeric and cumin.
  - Greek oregano and garlic stews.

· Mexican chili-lime blends.
· Middle Eastern za'atar with thyme, sesame, and sumac.

These aren't just recipes — they are longevity practices.

Myth-Busting Herbs & Spices
Myth #1: "They're just flavoring."

Wrong. Herbs and spices are concentrated medicine. The compounds that make them taste strong — like allicin in garlic or curcumin in turmeric — are the same compounds that regulate immunity, block tumor growth, and reduce inflammation.

Myth #2: "They don't matter if you already eat plants."

False. While fruits and vegetables provide fiber, vitamins, and minerals, herbs and spices add unique phytochemicals not found elsewhere. For example: curcumin (turmeric), cinnamaldehyde (cinnamon), and capsaicin (chili peppers) are distinct compounds with unique benefits.

Myth #3: "More salt equals more flavor."

No. Salt numbs taste buds. Herbs and spices awaken them. Over time, reducing salt and increasing herbs enhances flavor sensitivity, letting you enjoy food more — while protecting your heart and kidneys.

Myth #4: "They're too small to matter."

Completely false. Science shows even 1 teaspoon of cinnamon daily improves insulin sensitivity. A clove of garlic can drop blood pressure. A pinch of turmeric reduces inflammation markers. Small doses, repeated consistently, matter immensely.

Expanded Key Takeaways

- Herbs and spices are **concentrated medicine** in small packages.
- Turmeric, garlic, ginger, rosemary, cinnamon, and oregano protect against cancer.
- Spices ease ailments like high blood sugar, pain, and poor digestion.
- Salt is the exception — keep intake under 1,200 mg/day.
- Replacing salt with herbs and spices builds flavor and healing simultaneously.
- Cultural longevity traditions prove: herbs and spices are daily, not optional.
- Science validates what ancient wisdom already knew — food is medicine, and herbs are its strongest dose.

Action Steps

1. Replace salt with at least one herb or spice at every meal.
2. Add turmeric and black pepper to one dish daily.
3. Drink a cup of herbal tea — ginger, cinnamon, hibiscus, or peppermint.
4. Keep fresh garlic on hand and use it raw or lightly cooked daily.
5. Rotate spices weekly — aim for at least five different herbs/spices daily.
6. Journal your meals for a week — note how energy, digestion, or mood shifts when you add healing spices.

Closing Message

Herbs and spices may look small, but their impact is profound. They fight cancer, reverse ailments, lower blood pressure, regulate blood sugar, and allow you to live with flavor instead of fear.

The truth is simple: **season with healing.**

In *The P53 Diet & Lifestyle,* I highlighted how garlic, turmeric, and ginger shift the terrain toward resilience. In *Taste Versus Cancer,* I showed how phytochemicals in herbs and spices block tumor growth and repair DNA.

This book brings the message full circle: **keep salt down, keep flavor up, and let every meal be a prescription for life.**

When you embrace herbs and spices, you realize that medicine doesn't come in bottles. It comes in sprigs, roots, powders, and seeds. They may be the smallest ingredients in the kitchen — but they are the biggest allies in your health.

Chapter 19

Taking Back Control: How to Own Your Health

For most of modern history, people have been told that health comes from outside themselves — from doctors, drugs, supplements, or "miracle" cures in glossy packages. But throughout this book, we've stripped away the illusions. We've seen how:

- Deficiencies weaken the body silently until disease takes hold.
- Animal products burden health with hormones, cholesterol, and cancer-promoting compounds.
- Pills and supplements mask symptoms while draining nutrients.
- Processed foods overload the body with sugar, oils, and chemicals.
- Exercise builds resilience — but only when paired with the right fuel.
- And how herbs and spices, often overlooked, amplify healing by reducing inflammation, balancing blood sugar, and even blocking cancer pathways.

The truth is simple: the power was never out there. The power has always been inside you — in the choices you make daily, in the foods you eat, in how you move, rest, breathe, and season your life.

The Core Message of This Book

If you take only one thing away from everything you've read, let it be this:

Your body wants to heal. Your choices decide whether it can.

- Fill it with whole plant foods, and it thrives.
- Move daily, and it grows stronger.
- Rest deeply, and it resets and rebuilds.
- Breathe, manage stress, and your hormones rebalance.
- Remove toxins, and the pathways of repair open.
- Add herbs and spices, and you supercharge your terrain — reducing inflammation, stabilizing blood sugar, and defending against DNA damage.

Health is not complicated. It's not expensive. It's a return to simplicity.

The Hard Truth

No doctor can exercise for you.

No pill can eat vegetables for you.

No supplement can sprinkle turmeric or garlic on your food for you.

No prescription can stop you from pouring salt into your arteries.

Only you can do those things. And when you do, the body responds with healing, energy, clarity, and resilience. That is the hard truth — but also the most empowering truth.

Your Daily Power

You don't need a complex protocol or expensive gadgets. You don't need 50 supplements in the cabinet. You don't need to chase trends or buy into gimmicks. What you need is daily power — consistent habits that nourish your terrain.

The Eight Pillars of Daily Ownership
1. Start the Day with Plants

Fruit for breakfast. Oats with flaxseed. Smoothies with spinach, banana, and berries. The way you start your day sets your chemistry for the next 12 hours.

2. Move Every Day

Your ancestors walked, carried, climbed, and stretched. You don't need a marathon. You need motion. Even a brisk 30-minute walk rewires metabolism, boosts mood, and strengthens immunity.

3. Hydrate and Cleanse

Water is the cheapest detox. Replace soda, juice, and energy drinks with water, herbal teas, or sparkling water with lemon. Hydration flushes toxins instead of recirculating them.

4. Anchor Meals in Beans and Greens

Build every plate around legumes, vegetables, and whole grains. Beans stabilize blood sugar, greens provide calcium and antioxidants, and whole grains deliver sustained energy.

5. Keep Salt Low, Flavor High

Salt kills silently. Keep sodium under **1,200 mg/day.** Replace it with herbs and spices: garlic, turmeric, cinnamon, oregano, basil, ginger, rosemary, cumin. Every pinch is not just flavor — it's protection.

6. Rest and Rebuild

Healing happens at night. Prioritize 7–9 hours of sleep, free of late-night meals and blue light. Sleep is the most underrated medicine on Earth.

7. Listen to Symptoms as Signals

Your body whispers before it screams. Fatigue, headaches, rashes, bloating — they're not random. They are teachers. Instead of silencing them with pills, ask: **What is this trying to tell me?**

8. Keep Toxins Out

Stop pouring poisons into the terrain. Avoid ultra-processed food, refined sugar, toxic oils, and chemical preservatives like sodium benzoate. Cut fluoride, aluminum, and dyes. Every toxin removed frees your immune system to do its real job: protection.

Herbs and Spices: The Finishing Touch

Think of herbs and spices as amplifiers.

- Turmeric turns down inflammation pathways.
- Garlic detoxifies and lowers blood pressure.
- Cinnamon stabilizes sugar and protects against cancer.
- Rosemary and oregano sharpen immunity and defend DNA.
- Ginger calms pain and improves digestion.

Sprinkled daily, they multiply the effects of your plant-based foundation. They are not garnish. They are medicine.

Final Closing Message

Stories of Hope

I've seen people reverse diabetes by trading pills for plants, salt for spices, and fear for ownership.

I've seen heart patients drop blood pressure not with drugs, but with garlic, flaxseed, and beans.

I've seen cancer survivors build resilience by seasoning every meal with turmeric, ginger, and cruciferous vegetables.

I've seen hopeless people regain joy when they realized health was not lost — it was waiting for them in their daily choices.

Final Key Takeaways

- **You are not powerless.**
- **Whole plants, herbs, movement, rest, and toxin reduction are your true medicine.**
- **Pills manage disease; lifestyle prevents and heals it.**
- **Health isn't a product. It's a practice.**

The Final Truth

Your body is not your enemy. It is your ally. It wants to heal, repair, and thrive.

The truth is simple: **you are in control. Always have been. Always will be.** The only question is whether you will use that power.

In ***The P53 Diet & Lifestyle,*** I laid out the science of plant-based healing. In ***Taste Versus Cancer,*** I showed how cancer is not random but rooted in terrain. In my research on pharmaceuticals and supplements, I revealed how the very drugs people rely on often deplete the nutrients they need most.

This book has simplified the message: **plants, herbs, and lifestyle are medicine. Pills are not.**

Herbs and spices are the smallest things in your kitchen, but they may be the biggest reminders of truth: that health is flavor, color, variety, and life.

So season your life wisely. Move with intention. Rest deeply. Eat plants. Listen to your body. Keep toxins out.

Because in the end, health was never in the pill bottle. It was always in your hands. I hope the information in this book can give you a healthier life. For more information on health & nutrition please visit my website thep53.com.

For those of you that need one on one coaching help please contact Truett Standefer by visiting www.lumen8life.com.